THE NEW REVISED
SIXTH AND SEVENTH
BOOKS OF MOSES

AND

THE MAGICAL USES OF THE PSALMS

THE NEW REVISED

SIXTH AND SEVENTH

BOOKS OF MOSES

AND

THE MAGICAL USES OF THE PSALMS

EDITED BY

MIGENE GONZÁLEZ-WIPPLER

This book was first published in Stuttgart, Germany in 1849 under the title, Das Sechste und Siebente Buch Mosis. The first American edition published in New York in 1880.

First revised edition published in 1982.
Second edition published in 1991.

ISBN 0-942272-02-1

THE SIXTH AND SEVENTH
BOOKS OF MOSES

THE MYSTERY OF ALL MYSTERIES

The Citation On All Spirits, The Spirit In The Burning
Bush, "Helmet of Moses And Aaron,"
Healing By Amulets

THE WONDERFUL MAGICAL AND
SPIRIT ARTS

Of Moses And Aaron, And The Old Wise Hebrews, Taken From
The Mosaic Books Of The Cabala And The Talmud,
For The Good Of Mankind

RARE OLD MOSAIC BOOKS OF THE TALMUD AND CABALA

Contains
One Hundred and Twenty-Five
Seals and Talismans

*Translated From The German Original, Word For Word,
according To The Old Ancient Writings and
Famous Manuscripts of the Hebrews.*

With exact copies of over One Hundred and Twenty-Five
Seals, Signs, Emblems, etc., used by Moses, Aaron, Israelites,
Egyptians, etc., in their astounding Magical and other Arts,
including the period of time covered by the Old and New
Testaments. This wonderful translation is of great importance to the student of Occultism. The extracts from the old
and rare Mosaic Books of the Talmud and Cabala are invalu-
able. The book contains 125 illustrations which are exact
copies of the stone tablets used by the Israelites and Egyptians
to accomplish their designs for good or evil, and are sepa-
rately explained.

Contents

Preface to the Revised Edition

The Sixth and Seventh Books of Moses was originally published in Stuttgart, Germany, in 1849. Its author, a German author by the name of Johann Scheibel, is shrouded in mystery. Public records indicate that he was born in 1736 and died in 1809, forty years before the publication date of the present work. This would seem to indicate that the book was published posthumously, but there are no indications as to who was responsible for the 1849 publication. Scheibel wrote several books in his lifetime, including a biographical work and an astronomical treatise. To complicate matters further some sections of the book are dated as far back as 1338, 1383 and 1501, with indications that they were translated into English, not from the German language, but from the "Cuthan-Samaritan." The language used in the original version is largely archaic, and had to be rewritten in several instances.

The author claimed that the seals and invocations given in the book came from ancient Hebrew sources, particularly the Talmud. It is not sure whether or not his claims were based on truth, although Talmudic scholars will probably deny that there are any references in Talmudic literature to the Sixth and Seventh Books of Moses.

While the original source of the book will probably never be ascertained, its popularity and durability can hardly be denied. This revised edition is an attempt at the reorganization of a work, long hailed by occult masters as a valuable tool in the study and practice of Kabbalistic magic.

Nothing has been added to the original material, with the exception of short explanatory notes where they seemed necessary. Also the reorganization of the text has made it necessary to transpose material from some sections to others. Some editing has been done on parts of the work that were unclear, or whose archaic language made it difficult to understand. But every effort has been made to adhere to the original text whenever possible. For example, whenever Latin and English have been mixed in the text, the editor has resisted most temptations to edit. Neither has any attempt been made to correct some of the Hebrew names which have been undoubtedly corrupted during translation and subsequent editions. All invocations and seals have been reproduced intact.

The quaint language of the work has been left untouched for the most part, with some minor editorial changes. It must be remembered that some parts of this work date as far back as the Sixteenth Century, and to alter the language extensively would be to risk losing the true meaning intended by the original author and the translator. And although some of the written text may seem at times Pontifical and dogmatic in the extreme, there is enough wisdom hidden throughout the work to warrant the most careful reading on the part of the discerning reader.

It is hoped that this new edition will make the teachings of this venerable work attainable to many readers who up to now were unable to understand it. Undoubtedly, much of the material herein is of little value to the student because of its adulterated nature, but those who are able to glean the gold from the chaff will benefit vastly from this work. If they can fulfill this task, I will consider my humble efforts amply rewarded.

Migene González-Wippler

PART I

THE MAGIC OF THE ISRAELITES

(ABRIDGED)

The complete and reliable history of the human and divine — the divine revelations and the influence or pious men — are found in the Scriptural monuments of the old Hebrews, in the Holy Scriptures.

The Bible is called the Holy Scriptures because it contains knowledge of the saints, while at the same time it unites and harmonizes word and deed, doctrine and action. It points out the true relation of man to the Omnipotent, that is, it provides the most direct reference to the great truths of the spiritual and the intellectual; it discourses on the origin of the universe and its laws (through which all things come into being), on the beginning and the end of mankind, on man's destiny and how he may attain it, on the living and visible agents which God employs in the great work of redemption, and finally, on the most exalted of all beings, the World's Savior, who was a universal expression in himself, and who exhibited all divine power and action in one person, while all his forerunners were endowed only with limited powers. It was he who revealed to a fallen mankind the highest and purest ideals, the divine purpose of life, and the means of purification and restoration.

We find among oriental nations every aspect of magic. Although these are also present among the Israelites, they are totally different in character. In other nations, it was the individual who mattered. In Israel, the emphasis was placed on mankind and upon mankind's future. In other nations, the light of man was made to shine by skillful actions, by the lowest arts. In Israel, there shown a pure unclouded light, vitalized by the breath of the Almighty, a light shining into the future, a light upon which depended all light and action. To the Israelite seer, not only the fate of single individuals stands revealed, but also the fate of nations, of mankind, which in the end must be reconciled to God by the unfolding of magical art, as often happened under the old dispensation by instinctive sonambulistic influences. If we examine the history of the old covenant, we find that this remarkable people stood solitary, like a pillar of fire amid heathen darkness.

Although we find among other nations worthy men who seek after the divine light, surrounded by darkness and uncertainty, in

Israel we find men of God bearing the seal of true faith, who give undoubted evidence of higher powers by visible acts and signs which separate life from death and truth from error. While the ancient remnants of other nations show only theory without application, in Israel we find a connected chain of acts and events, in fact, a divine and life-like drama. Of all these things the various books of Holy Scriptures speak with confidence so that the history of no other people interwovern with fables can be compared with them. According to this, the Bible contains the light which illuminates every dark phase of life. It is the groundwork of all human actions, the guiding star of the earthly to the eternal, of the intellectual to the divine, the aim and end of all knowledge.

The Bible is also more instructive and richer than all other books taken together. For example, the dreams recorded in the Bible are many and remarkable. The voice with which God spoke to the prophets and the men consecrated to Him, was generally heard in dreams. Numbers 12'6, Job 33'15, I Kings 3:5, Genesis 20:3, 31:23, and 37:5 are only a few Bible citations where the prophetic quality of dreams is exalted. But God sometimes spoke directly to some chosen men, like Moses and Jesus.

Let us look at the history of creation, as recorded by Moses in Genesis. "In the beginning God created heaven and earth..." Herein lies the first Cause, God is an uncreated being. Heaven and earth are the first things created, that is, the antithesis, that which was made of God. In reference to a second antithesis, Moses speaks of light and darkness: "And darkness was upon the face of the earth, and God said, Let there be light, and there was light." This concerns light as a creation with darkness as its opposite. The ancient Egyptians regarded darkness as the beginning of all things. But although the Egyptian doctrine in its first inception may be regarded as good authority, they erred in their belief that darkness came before the light. The Persians, who claimed that the light came before darkness, also erred. In reality, light stands beside darkness as its natural opposite. "And God divided the light from the darkness, and God called the light day, and the darkness he called night."

The Bible also points out another antithesis in water and spirit. "And the spirit of God moved upon the face of the waters." The water is matter, the germ of the figurative; the spirit - the Elohim - is the fruitful, active principle. One-sided views led earlier philosophers into numerous errors. For example, Thales believed everything came out of the water, thus overlooking the spiritual active whole. Subsequent champions of materialism followed his lead, also missing the obvious. on the opposite side wr. the advocates of Spiritualism, who preached that everything is spirit, matter being only an inert abstraction. Moses showed his superiority over all the disciples of Egyptian-temple wisdom, as well as over the more modern sects, inasmuch as he was enlightened by divine wisdom and ascribed to matter its true worth, placing it side by side with the spirit.

The Mosaic Eden was the habitation of purely created beings, within whose boundaries grew the tree of knowledge of good and evil. The serpent is a symbol of fallen man. What follows in this context comes from a mystical manuscript, entitled, Magikon, or, The Secret System of an Association of Unknown Philosophers, v. 27-31, published in Frankfurt and Leipzig in 1784.

"In view of his divine origin, as an unconditional emanation from God, Adam was an expression of divine power. He was a heavenly being brought into existence by God himself and was not born into the world like ordinary men. He also enjoyed, because of his divine nature, all the prerogatives of a pure spirit, surrounded by an invulnerable veil. But his was not a physical body, which he gained only as an evidence of his degradation — a course mantle — by which he sought to protect himself against the raging elements. His garments were holy, simple, indestructible, and of an indissoluble character. He was created in this condition of perfect glory, in which he enjoyed the purest happiness, in order to reveal the power of the Almighty and to ensure that he would rule over the visible and the invisible. As the symbol of unity, he was safe from the attacks of all enemies because the veil by which he was covered (the germs of which are still in us), rendered him invulnerable."

Christ promised the same invulnerability to his apostles and to all his followers through the regeneration of man. In this condition man also bears a fiery, double-edged sword, which is a living word, combining in itself all power, and through which "everything is possible to him." Of this sword, Moses says in Genesis 3:24, "So he drove out man, and he placed at the east end of the garden of Eden Cherubims, and a flaming sword which turned every way, to keep the tree of life." In Revelations 1:16, we read, "And out of his mouth went a two-edged sword." This sword represents the living word, which was originally inherent in man, and which can only be restored to him by his return to a pure state, and by being cleansed from his present state of sensualism. It is the word of which we read in Hebrews 4:12, "For the word of God is quick and powerful and sharper than a two-edged sword, piercing even to the dividing asunder of soul and spirit."

Among the most extraordinary words of power is the all-conquering **Honover** of Zoroaster, by means of which Ormuzd overcame Ahriman and all evil. "In this condition of kingly honor and power," we read further in the Magikon manuscript, "man could have enjoyed the purest happiness had he properly guarded his Eden, but he erred in confusing light with truth, and in so doing he lost both. Because he thought that he could find the light in another place, other than the first great fountain, he became involved in a false existence, grew enamored of sensualism, thus becoming sensual himself. Through this adultery he sank into darkness and confusion and now he experienced a sensual nakedness of which he was ashamed. Through this sin man lost, not only his original habitation, but also the "fiery sword," and with it everything else that made him all-seeing and unconquerable. His holy garments now became as the skin of animals, and this mortal, perishable covering afforded him no protection against the elements. With the wasted half of his body, the spiritual also added to the confusion, and discordant sounds were heard in the dark places of his spiritual domain."

Although man had sunk deep in sin, the hope of a full restoration was given to him on condition of perfect reconciliation with the Deity. Without such reconciliation, however, he sinks deeper and deeper in his own degradation, and his return becomes still more precarious. In order to be reconciled, he must become self-abased, and resist the false allurements of the material world, which only serve to steep him in the mire of the elements. Therefore he must seek, by means of prayer, to obtain the more exalted blessings of benevolent influences, without which he cannot draw a pure breath. In this reconciliation he must gradually overcome all, and put away everything that could destroy his inner nature and separate him from the great source of his being. He can never enjoy peace within himself and with nature around him until he has overcome everything opposed to his own nature, and gained victory over his enemies. This can only be done when he returns to the same road from which he wandered away. The following is a genuine extract from scriptural doctrine according to the Indian creed, differing, however, in character:

"The Almighty has provided means to aid man in the work of reconciliation. God has appointed higher agents to lead man back from the errors of his ways. But man can only be restored to this state of purity through the Saviour of the world, who finished and perfected all that these agents had accomplished only in part at different times. Through him all power became animated and exalted; through him, man approaches the only true light, a knowledge of all things, and, especially, a knowledge of himself. If man is willing to accept this offered help, he will arrive at the desired goal, and he will be so firmly established in faith that no future doubts can ever cause him to waver again. If he elevates his will so that it will be in unison with the divine will, he can spiritualize his being while still in this world until the spiritual kingdom becomes visible to his eyes and he can feel God nearer to him than he ever thought possible. In this state all things will become possible for him because he adds all power to his own, and in this union and harmony, with a fullness of a higher vitality, the divine agents, such as Moses, Elias, and even Christ himself may become visible to him. In short, man can attain such a degree of perfection, even in this life, that all death will mean to him will be a disrobing of his coarse covering to reveal his spiritual temple. His spiritual being will taste nobler fruits, and at the end of his race nothing will separate him from the exalted harmonies of those spheres, of

14

which mortal sense can draw but a faint picture. He will live the life of the angels and will possess all their powers. He will not only enjoy his own gifts, but will also share in the gifts of the elect, who constitute the council of the wise."

Let us now look at some of the remarkable magical occurrences related by the Bible. For example, the magnetic influence which results in the changing of the nature and the essence of living objects is seen in the history of Jacob. According to the Bible, Jacob agreed with Laban that he would guard Laban's sheep, provided that Laban would reward Jacob for this service by letting him keep all the ringed and spotted lambs and goats that should be born in the future. Laban agreed to this proposal. According to the story, which is related in Genesis 30:27-43, Jacob became immensely rich as a result of this agreement. This he accomplished through the magic known as "magnetic influence." How did he do this? Simply by taking thin reeds of the green poplar, hazel and chestnut trees, marking notches in them until the white bark appeared, thus creating an effect of streaks and spots on the bark. These marked reeds he placed inside the water troughs the cattle drank from. He only used the reeds when the cattle were strong, never when they were weak. When the cattle conceived after staring at the marked reeds through the water, they brought forth spotted, speckled, and streaked young. This Jacob kept for himself as he had agreed with Laban. The end result of this was that the best and the strongest cattle eventually became Jacob's property, while the weakest remained Laban's. And in time Jacob became so rich in cattle that Laban had to end the agreement and let Jacob go, which was what Jacob wanted all along.

This shows that the sheep and the goats could be made to conceive their young spotted and speckled simply by staring at spotted and speckled reeds. This theory which would be considered absurd today, finds some backing in the fact that the mental and physical quality of many children differ totally from those of their parents. Did Jacob know from experience that his stratagem would succeed or was it revealed to him in a dream? Genesis 31:10 says, "And it came to pass at the time the cattle conceived, that I lifted up mine eyes, and saw in a dream, and behold, the rams which leaped upon the cattle were ring-streaked, speckled and grizzled." With the water from which the cattle drank, and in which at the same time they saw their own reflection, they transmitted the image of the speckled reeds to their young. We have not the space here to enter into a more detailed argument to prove the truth of this phenomenon, but the fact that the female progenitor, both human and animal, is capable during the period of gestation to transmit to her offspring the image and likeness of surrounding objects, has a stronger foundation than is commonly believed to be possible.

Another Biblical instance resembling magnetism is the rod with which Moses performed his wonders before Pharoah and his court, and which he also used to divide the waters of the sea and to bring forth water from the rock at Rephidim. Moses used the rod in conjunction with the extending forth of his hand, and by the use of both he performed incredible feats. The magnetic power of the human hand is accepted even in our present time, and when this natural magnetism is multiplied by an unshakable faith and God-given powers, such as Moses had, the result can be awesome. The rod which Moses used was probably both a conductor and magnifier of his power, as well as a direct connection with God. When Amalek came to fight against Israel, Moses said to Joshua (Numbers 11:23-29), "Choose us out men, and go out, fight with Amalek; tomorrow I will stand on the top of the hill with the rod of God in my hand. And it came to pass, when Moses held up his hand, that Israel prevailed; and when he let down his hand, Amalek prevailed."

The gift of prophecy seems to have been given also to the pious elders of Israel through their relationship with Moses, for it is written in Numbers 11:23-29, "And the Lord said unto Moses, Is the Lord's hand waxed short? thou shalt see now whether my word shall come to pass unto thee or not. And Moses went out and told the people the words of the Lord, and gathered together the seventy men of the elders of the people, and set them around about the tabernacle. And the Lord came down in a cloud, and spake unto him and took the spirit that was upon him, and gave it unto the seventy elders: and it came to pass, that, when the spirit rested upon them, they prophesied and did not cease. But there remained two of the men in the camp, the name of the one was Eldad, and the name of the other Meldad: and the spirit rested upon them: and they were of them that were written, but went not out into the tabernacle: and they prophesied in the camp. And Joshua, the son of Nun, the servant of Moses, one of his young men, answered and said, My Lord Moses, forbid them. And Moses said unto him, Enviest thou for my sake? would God that all the Lord's people were prophets, and that the Lord would put his spirit in them!"

The personal conversations of God with Moses, and his power of beholding the Almighty in his true similitude are figurative expressions, and must not be taken in a literal sense. For the Lord speaks through revelation and by means of the light, and not by word of mouth; neither can God be seen by mortal eyes, for He says in another place, "No man can behold me and live." This language is the impression or expression of the divine word and a light from the purest source; it is the spiritual gift and revelation of the Deity to man, which must be taken according to the various grades of intelligence of beings, as in nature, according to the various grades of intelligence of beings, as in nature, according to the kind of light produced by different actions, whether the effect be produced upon near or distant objects.

The visions and prophecies of Balaam, the son of Beor, to whom Balak sent messengers so that he would curse Israel, are also of a remarkable character. In Numbers 24, we find a detailed account of the power of the heathen seer. It seems that Balak, king of the Moabites, being afraid of the Israelites, decided to form a league with the Midianites. But since neither the Moabites nor the Midianites felt like engaging in hostilities with the Israelites, they resorted to magic. Since they had no magician among themselves, they sent for Balaam, who was celebrated for his powers of charming and divining. The messengers came to Balaam with costly presents, and demanded that he should curse this strange people. Balaam invited them to tarry overnight. In the morning he arose and made known to the messengers that God neither permitted him to curse the Israelites, nor allowed him to accompany them to their country, for "that people was favored of God." Balak, thinking he had not offered enough, sent more costly presents to Balaam with his nobles, in order to induce the seer to visit him and curse Israel. Balaam, a mixture of faith and fickleness, of truth and avarice, of true prophecy and magic, said to the servants of Balak: "If Balak would give me his house full of silver and gold, I cannot go beyond word of the Lord my God, to do less or more." And yet, after he had spoken with the Lord during the night, he arose in the morning, saddled his ass, and prepared to go with the Moabite princes, and afterward told the enemies of Israel how they could lead Israel into idolatry.

"And God's anger was kindled against him because he went: and the angel of the Lord stood in his way for an adversary against him." The ass, with characteristic stubborness, preferred the field to the uneven paths in the vineyards, and when force was used to turn her in the way, she thrust herself against the wall, and crushed Balaam's foot against it, for which he smote her with his staff. Since there was no path to turn aside either to the right or to the left, the ass fell down under Balaam, and he smote her again. Finally the ass spoke to Balaam and pointed out to him his unreasonable conduct, and when Balaam heard this he beheld the angel of God, instead of the ass. Conscience-strickened, he confessed his sin and promised to go back whence he came, but the angel permitted him to proceed only upon condition that he should speak only what the Lord had commanded him to say. He fulfilled this condition in spite of every temptation that Balak could offer; and he went not at other times to seek for enchantments, but he set his face toward the wilderness. Instead of cursing the Israelites, he blessed them, and afterward actually prophesied concerning the Star of Jacob.

Among all the prophets of the Old Testament, the most exalted was Elias, whose very name was a symbol of high spirituality. In his many magical prowesses, we find great examples of magnetic transferences. He imparted the most important doctrines of life, and he gave life to such as had apparently died, as in the following story, related in I Kings 17:17-25. "And it came to pass after these things, that the son of the woman, the mistress of the house, fell sick, and his sickness was so sore, that there was no breath left in him. And she said unto Elias, what have I to do with thee, O thou man of God? art thou come unto me to call my sin to remembrance, and to slay my son? And he said unto her, Give me thy son. And he took him out of her bosom, and carried him up into a loft, where he abode, and laid him upon his own bed. And he cried unto the Lord, and said, O Lord, my God, hast thou also brought evil upon the widow with whom I sojourn, by slaying her son? And he stretched himself upon the child three times, and cried unto the Lord and said, O Lord, my God, I pray thee, let this child's soul come into him again, and he revived. And Elias took the child, and brought him down out of the chamber into the house, and delivered him to his mother."

The prophet Elisha also restored life, as it is related in II Kings 4:18-37. In that story Elisha restores the life of the Shunammite's son. Upon learning that the child was dead, Elisha sent his servant Gehazi ahead of him to the Shunamite's house, with Elisha's staff in his hand. He instructed Gehazi not to salute anyone in the street, and not to return any greetings that were proferred him while on his way. He was to lay Elisha's staff upon the child's face upon arrival at the Shunammite's house. But the child did not return to life with this action, and Elisha came himself to the house. He prayed unto the Lord, then stretched himself upon the child until the child's flesh "waxed warm." Elisha stood up, walked up and down the room several times, then stretched himself upon the child once more, who, this time sneezed seven times and opened his eyes to his mother's delight.

This story teaches us that true power comes from God. It also teaches us that Elisha knew how to transfer his power to another person - in this case, Gehazi - who acted as a conductor of the power. Elisha's power was concentrated on his staff, similar to the rod of Moses, but obviously Gehazi could not wield it with the same strength as Elisha's for the child did not return to life with Gehazi's ministrations. Elisha also knew that concentration is vital in magnetic magic, for he instructed Gehazi not to greet anyone along the way, obviously not to disperse his magical power. Perseverance and continuity are also important lessons in this story, for the child did not revive the first time Elisha lay down over him. Walking up and down the room served to recharge Elisha's psychic energies, which he used successfully to revive the boy in his second try. So powerful were Elisha's magical powers, that a man who was buried in Elisha's sepulchre came back to life as soon as his body touched Elisha's remains. This extraordinary resurrection is told in II Kings 13:20.

Prophetic inspiration is not a creation of nature or of man, but an emanation of the Holy Spirit and divine decree. The divine call comes unexpectedly, and the physical condition has no connection with it whatsoever. Physical powers can never become permanent powers, but always remain dependent upon the spirit. Magnetic second-sight, on the other hand, depends directly upon the health and life of the seer, or rather, it predominates in human life under certain circumstances. The clairvoyant directs his attention to specially selected objects, which he then analyzes with his clair- voyant powers; interprets his own visions or those other people bring to him. Purely human nature is very much within the magic circle of the seer, and the operation of his will and his faith produces no supernatural or permanent effect, either upon himself or upon others.

On the other hand, the prophet is not only a seer, but the executor of the divine will. Instruction in the true knowledge of God, and spreading his kingdom, which is truth and love, is the prophet's only interest. He therefore fights against error and wickedness, in an effort to overcome the world. He is not concerned with that which is worldly and changeable. Bigotry or sensuality, health, riches, and honor in the world, or dominion over his fellow men do not interest him. He does not preach a present, but a future state of happiness, genuine peace with God, and the hope of eternal life in His presence, not from personal impulse or selfish- ness, or from human considerations, but as a willing instrument of perpetual enlightenment, inspired by God Himself.

True prophets do not isolate themselves, neither do they sink into the absorbing depths of their own visions and feelings. Their prophecies do not refer to human personalities, but to the fate of nations and the world. They are therefore able to exhibit supernatural powers, strengthened by the omnipotent power of their faith and will, and they exercise this power over their own bodies, as well as over the bodies of others and over all of nature in its wide and temporal boundaries.

The prophetic and magical experiences of Israel, as recounted in the Bible, show that the causes of inward visions are actually objective, and that there is something outside of human intelligence that govens and controls the world of man independently of the inner centrum of the mind, while the peripheral sense of day and nature are either inactive, or in a very subordinate condition.

The Biblical narrative reveals also that there is a more exalted spiritual region which takes a positive hold upon the reason and offers revelations which are not of a natural order, and which are not merely fantasies of the brain.

According to the Bible, God has made use of the noblest of impulses of the spirit of Israel for the education and redemption of the human family, and that this people, who were disobedient and stubborn, could only be brought to face their true destiny by means of severe chastisement and adversity. To this people, and no other, were the commandments communicated in thunder tones by divinely appointed leaders, so that they might heed God's message with the inner depths of the mind and not superficially with the outward senses. Sacrifices and feasts were not to serve as temporal occasions of rejoicing, but as means to attain the revelation of the true light of the coming Messiah. The Mercy Seat, The Cherubim, the Holy of Holies, the Pillar of Fire, and Solomon's Temple, were all symbolical manifestations originating in magical visions, and pointed to the coming of Christ. The entire Mosaic experience was symbolical and hieroglyphical. Moses, the Man of God, constitutes in the history of the children of Israel the second period of the beginning of religious development, the first period being Abraham's convenant with God. The forms and ceremonies of the law were strictly enforced with Moses in order to impress upon mankind the importance of the revealed word. King David, with whom commenced the third period, solidified the foundations of Israel's inheritance, ratified the original covenant and united the twelve tribes of Israel into a mighty kingdom. This union, which was magical as well as physical, is exemplified in David's enduring symbol, the six-pointed star that bears his name.

Having discussed the old covenant at some length, it would seem proper also to discuss the new covenant, because it describes many instances of magical healings effected without visible means by Christ and the apostles. It would appear from these stories that all these miracles and healings were the result of magic or magnetism. The men of God who, under the old covenant performed such great wonders, and accomplished such wonderful works, were always more on the side of humanity that that of the divine. That is, they always evinced single powers and perfections. The universal expression of perfection became a reality only through Christ. It was he who first unbarred the new door, severed the chains of slavery, and pointed out the true images of perfection and wisdom to mankind. Christ restored to humanity the assurance of immortality. He elevated the spiritual being to a temple of holy fire, and made it a living altar and incense to eternal peace.

The art of healing, according to scriptural principles, deserves special mention in this place, not only because something truly magical takes place therein, but because scriptural healing is often regarded as the only true healing. The principles of this art of healing have been fully established according to certain declarations and doctrines of the Bible (See Leviticus 26:14; Deuteronomy 28:15-22; Exodus 14:26; and Psalms 107:17-20).

In the New Testament diseases are generally ascribed to sin. Jesus said to the paralytic when he healed him:"Thy sins are forgiven thee," and he was made whole. And when he healed the man at the pool of Bethesda, who had an infirmity for thirty-eight years, when he met him afterward in the temple, he said to him: "Behold thou art made whole; sin no more, lest a greater evil befall thee." (John 5:14).

The apostles, too, and all the saints, insisted upon first curing the patient morally, for a true restoration of the diseased body and spirit can only be effected by a return to God. It is truly remarkable that he wise men of the East, Zoroaster, and all the advocates of the doctrines of emission (system of emanation), the Kabbalists, as well as later Theosophists, all of whom possessed extraordinary powers to heal diseases, defended this doctrine. Some of these men believed that diseases are caused by sin, while others attributed them to evil spirits, with whom men become associated through sin.

The originally pure doctrine of Christianity was prepared in early times by the advocates of the system of emanations, which was more destructive through misrepresentations by model Christians than was intended. Saturninus, Basilides and Karpokrates headed those who believed everything proceeded from the Aeon (heavenly powers). Christ himself was to them an Aeon of the first rank, who, by a rigid restraint from sensualism subdued demons (evil spirits), and he who lives as Christ did can subdue them likewise. "Out of Aeon, the chief outlet," said Basilides, heaven was brought into existence." According to Valentine, one of the most celebrated teachers of that day, the Aeons were divided into classes, such as male and female. Thus, the chief female Aeon was the Holy Sprit. By the laying of consecrated hands, the subject was made the recipient of this Aeon and was sent out to heal demoniac diseases. Although this digression created a variety of ideas differing from the original doctrine, the healing of diseases according to scriptural principles continued for a great length of time.

If a person is in earnest about living his life in unconditional obedience to God, and becomes converted to God through living, active faith, then God becomes his physician, and he no longer requires the services of an earthly doctor. As soon as the soul is in a perfectly healthy condition, this health will be communicated to the body. But if a person is not capable to heal himself through faith, then he must have recourse to a physician.

There are examples in the Bible where physical remedies were employed by some of the prophets. Moses, for example, by casting wood into the waters of Marah, made them sweet (Exodus 15:25). He cured leprosy by washing and purifying. Elias, on the other hand, threw salt into the bitter spring, and it became palatable afterwards. He also cast meal into the pot wherein was death, and the vegetables became harmless. Isaiah laid figs on the glands of King Hezekiah and healed him. Tobias cured his blind father with fishgall, a cure that was shown to him by an angel. Jesus himself anointed the eyes of the blind man with spittle and clay, and told him to wash in the pool of Siloam.

According to the Bible, only outward remedies were used in healing, and these of the simplest kinds. Internal remedies were not used. The means of cure consisted in spiritual purifications, in conversion from sin, in prayers to God, the believer's physician. So we read in James 5:13-16. "Is any among you afflicted? Let him pray. Is any merry? Let him sing psalms. Is any sick among you? Let him call the elders of the church, and let them pray over him, anointing him with oil in the name of the Lord."

But the scriptural physician does not always heal and the disease is not always evil. If temporal enjoyment and earthly joys were the destiny and the end of man, then should we be justified in regarding sickness as a great misfortune and a heavy punishment, which many will not admit of having deserved? This planet is not an abode of perfect peace and happiness. Light and darkness, night and day, love and hate, peace and war, life and death, are only some of the constant changes we face in this world. And they are not due to accident, but are arranged with meticulous care by a higher hand, so that we may, through affliction and suffering, overcome evil and purify ourselves from sensualism, thus preparing for a better existence. Our main objective should be the health of the soul and the spirit; the health of the body is a secondary matter. Because if the soul is in a state of radiant health, the body will reflect this health. "His flesh shall be fresher than a child's; he shall return to the days of his youth." (Job 33:25)

Because true peace and happiness cannot be found in this world, we should not mourn the evanescence of simple joys, the transitory quality of human love, the fragility of human life. All these things will lose importance if we accept that this world is an illusion, and that we will one day know the reality of true joys in another existence, in the true home of our souls.

Part II

THE SIXTH AND SEVENTH

BOOKS OF MOSES

EDITOR'S NOTE:

The Sixth and Seventh Books of Moses are a compilation of seals, tables and talismans with kabbalistic engravings, designed for the purpose of invoking the aid of angels and other powerful spirits, in all types of human endeavors.

The Seven Seals of the Spirits fall within the province of the Sixth Book, while the Twelve Tables of the Spirits are given as part of the Seventh Book. The General Citation and the Magical Circle, which follow immediately, are to be used in conjunction with the Seals and the Tables.

Before starting any of the invocations connected with any of the Seals or Tables, the would-be magician should trace a reasonable facsimile of the circle on the floor or on a piece of black material. The usual dimensions of a magical circle are nine feet in diameter. Oriens in the diagram means east, and those words should be facing in an eastern direction, as should the magician, all during the invocation. The simplest way to locate the east is to find where the sun rises in the morning.

The room where this ceremony takes place should be as clean as possible, and it should also be purified beforehand. A simple purification ritual would be to aspergate the room with salt water, and then to carry a censer through it with live coals upon which have been poured both frankincense and garlic skins. Most occult masters recommened sexual abstinence and total fast for 24 hours before the ceremony.

Either the Seal or the Table to be used should be traced on a piece of virgin parchment with dove's blood ink, a magical substance easily found in most occult shops. Plenty of frankincense (no garlic this time) and myrrh, or any other type of incense agreeable to the planetary spirits, should be burned during the ceremony. A white candle should be burned on a candlestick on each of the cardinal points of the circle. (Oriens=East; Meridiens=South; Occidens=West; Septemtry=North).

After finishing the invocation, the magician should mentally banish all spiritual influences from the room before leaving the circle and putting out the candles.

A short explanation must be inserted here about the meaing of Kabbalah and Kabbalistic magic. The Kabbalah is the esoteric doctrine of the ancient Hebrews. It is said to come from the Hebrew root Kibel, which means "to receive." Kabbalah is the magic taught to Moses by God and his angels, according to tradition. This secret teaching was passed on orally by Moses to Aaron and Joshua, and from them to succeeding generations of Hebrews. Its magic is based upon the mysteries of the Tree of Life.

It is not possible in a short explanation to discuss Kabbalah at length, and the interest readers are directed to several excellent works on the subject. Chief among these are the Kabbalah by Christian Ginsburg, The Holy Kabbalah by Edward Waite and The Mystical Qabalah by Dione Fortune. This editor has also written a book on the subject, entitled A Kabbalah for the Modern World.

The General Citation

NECROMANTIA, SEU MAGICA ALBA ET NIGRA TRANSLATED EX THORA XXTA BIBL. ARCAN

Aba, Jehovah, Agla, Aschaij, Chad, Yah, Saddaij, Vedreh, Aschre, Noosedu, Zawa, Agla. Here utter the names of the angels of the Seal or Table, and their proper names. Continue as follows:

Eheije, Aijscher, Eneije, Weatta, Eloheij, Harenij, Yechuateche, Hagedola, Merof, Zaroteij, Agla, Pedenij, Zije, Kotecha, Barach, Amijm, Gedolijm, Verachena, Aleij, Weijazijloti, Mijkol, Zara, Umikol, Ra, Schadaij, Jehovah, Adonai, Zeboath, Zah, Elohim, Yeasch, Jepfila, Vaij, Bearechet, Vaij, Yomar, Ahaha, Elohim, Ascher, Hithalleij, Chuabotheij, Lepha, Viaj, Yehuel.

Here stop for a short time in prayer to God. Surrender yourself into the will of Almighty God. He will conduct your undertaking to your best interest. Hereupon take again the Seal or the Table written on parchment in your hand, and begin anew the citation above. Should your desire still remain unfulfilled, continue as follows:

Hamneijs, Hakha, Elohim, Horro, Heotij, Meo, Dij, Adhaijijon, Hazze, Hamalach, Haggo, Elohij, Mijcol, Rhab, Yeba, Rech, Elhaneah, Tijmneik, Ka, Rebe, Hem, Sohemne, Schembotaij, Veischak, Vegid, Gulaooc, Kered, Haarez, Jeha. Since the effects and appearances will now follow, you wishes as fulfilled. Otherwise repeat the Citation Toties quoties (in full).

The Magical Operation is made within this Circle.

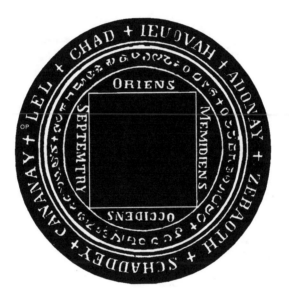

THE

Sixth Book of Moses.

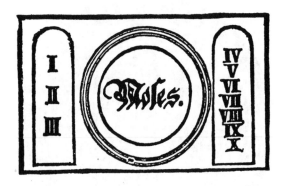

MOSES' MAGICAL SPIRIT-ART.

Translated from the Ancient Hebrew.

1. The Seven Seals of the Spirits

MAGIA ALBA ET NIGRA UNIVERSALIS SEU NECROMANTIA

That which embraces the whole of the White and Black Art (Black Magic), or the Necromancy of all Ministering Angels and Spirits; how to cite and desire the nine choruses of the good angels and spirits, Saturn, Jupiter, Mars, Sun, Venus, Mercury and Moon.

The most serviceable angels are SALATHEEL, MICHAEL, RAPHAEL, and URIEL, together with the Necromancy of the black magic of the best Ministering Spirits in the Chymia et Alchymia of Moses and Aaron.

That which was hidden from David, the father of Solomon, by the High Priest SADOCK, as the highest mystery, but which was finally found in the year 330 A.D., among others, by the first Christian Emperor Constantine the Great, and sent to Pope Sylvester at Rome, after its translation under Julius II, Pontifice Maximus. Typis Manabilis sub poena excommunications de numquam publica imprimendis sent to the Emperor Charles V, and highly recommended in the year 1520 A.D., approved By Pope Julius II, duos libros quos Mosis condidit arter antistis sedalitate SADOCK. Libri hi colorum sacra sunt vota sequenter spiritus omnipotens qui uigil illa facit at est sumis pia necessaria. Fides.

Instruction

These two books were revealed by God, the Almighty, to his faithful servant Moses, on Mount Sinai, intervale lucis, and in this manner they also came into the hands of Aaron, Caleb, Joshua, and Finally to David and his son Solomon, and their high priest, Sadock. Therefore, they are Bibliis arcanum arcanorum, which means Mystery of all Mysteries.

The Conversation of God

Adonai, Sother, Emanuel Ehic, Tetragrammaton, Ayscher, Jehova, Zebaoth, the Lord of Hosts, of Heaven and Earth; that which appertains to the Sixth and Seventh Books of Moses, as follows:

Adonai, E El, Zeboath, Jebaouha, Jehovah, E El, Chad, Tetragrammaton Chaddai, Channaniah, Al Elyon, Chaye, Ayscher, Adoyah Zawah, Tetragrammaton, Awiel, Adoyah, Chay, Yechal, Kanus, Emmet. Thus spake the Lord of Hosts to me Moses.

Eheye, Ayscher, Jehel, Yasliah, Elion. Sum qui sum ab aeterno in aeternum. Thou, my servant Moses, open thou thine ears, hear the voice of thy God. Through me Jehovah, Aglai, the God of heaven and earth, thy race shall be multiplied and shall shine as the stars of heaven. In addition to this, I will also give thee might, power and wisdom, to rule over the spirits of heaven and hell.

Over the ministering angels and spirits of the fourth element as well as of the seven planets. Hear also the voice of thy God wherewith I give thee the seven seals and twelve tables. Schem, Schel, Hamforach, that the angels and spirits may always yield obedient service to thee, when thou callest upon them and citest them by these seven seals and twelve tables of my omnipotence; and whereunto thou shalt also have herewith a knowledge of the highest mysteries.

Therefore, thou, my faithful friend, dear Moses, take thou the power and high might of thy God.

Aclon, Ysheye, Channanyah, E El, Elijon, Rachmiel, Ariel, Eheye, Ayscher, Eheye, Elyon. Through my seals and tables.

EDITOR'S NOTE:

The preceding information is given to the reader so that he knows that according to magical tradition the Sixth and Seventh Books of Moses, the Seals and the Tables within, were revealed by God to Moses on Mount Sinai. The section called **The Conversation of God** is enclosed, so he knows the words allegedly used by The Almighty to make this revelation unto Moses. None of this material is to be used during the invocations, either for the Seals or the Tables.

Of the information given with each seal, only the conjuration is to be used during the ceremony. The information that appears underneath each seal is descriptive of the seal and instructs the reader and would-be magician on the uses of each seal.

THE MYSTERY OF THE FIRST SEAL
Seal of the Choir of the Ministering Archangels
Conjuration

I, N.N.*, a servant of God, desire, call upon the OCH, and conjure thee through water, fire, air and earth, and everything that lives and moves therein, and by the most holy names of God, Agios, Tehirios, Perailitus, Alpha et Omega, Beginning and End, God and Man-Sabaoth, Adonai, Agla, Tetragrammaton, Emanuel, Abua, Ceus, Elioa, Torna, Deus Salvator, Aramma, Messias, Clerob, Michael, Abreil, Achleof, Gachenas et Peraim, Eei Patris et Peraim Eei filii, et Peraim Dei spiritus Teti, and the words by which Solomon and Manases, Cripinus and Agrippa conjured the spirits, and by whatever else thou mayest be conquered, that you will yield obedience to me, N.N.*, the same as Isaac did to Abraham, and appear before me, N.N.* this instant, in the beautiful, mild, human form of a youth, and bring what I desire. (This the conjuror must name.)

The First Seal

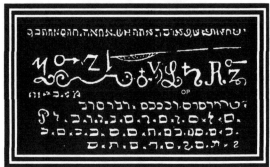

Fig. 2

The most useful ministering archangels of this seal are the following with their Hebrew verbis revelatis Citatiori divinitus coactivitis: Uriel, Arael, Zacharael, Gabriel, Raphael, Theoska, Zywolech, Hemohon, Yhahel, Tuwahel, Donahan, Sywaro, Samohayl, Zowanus, Ruweno, Ymoeloh, Hahowel, Tywael. The particularly great secret and special use of this seal is that if this seal is buried in the earth where treasures exist, they will come to the surface of themselves during a full moon.

*Whenever the initials N.N. appear in any of the seals, tables or invocations, the conjuror must substitute the initials with his full name.

THE MYSTERY OF THE SECOND SEAL

The Name is True
Seal of the Choir of Hosts or Dominations of the Ministering Angels

Conjuration

I, N.N., a servant of God, desire, call upon and conjure thee, Spirit Phuel, by the Holy Messengers and all the Disciples of the Lord, by the Four Holy Evangelists and the three Holy Men of God and by the most terrible and most holy words Abriel, Fibriel, Zada, Zarabo, Laragola, Lavaterium, Laroyol, Zay, Zagin, Labir, Lya, Adeo, Deus, Alon, Abay, Alos, Pieus, Ehos, Mibi, Uini, Mora, Zorad, and by those holy words, that thou come and appear before me, N.N., in a beautiful human form, and bring me what I desire. (This the conjuror must name.)

The Second Seal

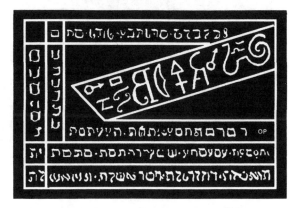

Fig. 3

This Seal from the Choir of Dominations or Hosts names the following spirits as the most useful: Aha, Roah, Habu, Aromicha, Lemar, Patteny, Hamaya, Azoth, Hayozer, Karohel, Wezinna, Patecha, Tehom. The special secret of this Seal is that if a man carries this Seal with him, it will bring him great fortune and blessings; it is therefore call the truest and highest Seal of fortune.

THE MYSTERY OF THE THIRD SEAL

Seal of the Ministering Throne Angels

Conjuration

I, N.N., a servant of God, desire, call upon thee, and conjure thee, by all the Holy Angels and Archangels, by the holy Michael, the holy Gabriel, Raphael, Uriel, Thrones, Principal Dominations, Virtues, Cherubim and Seraphim, and with unceasing voice I cry, Holy, Holy, Holy, is the Lord God Sabaoth, and by the most terrible words: Soab, Sother, Emmanuel, Hdon, Amathon, Mathay, Adonai, Eel, Eli, Eloy, Zoag, Dios, Anath, Tafa, Uabo, Tetragrammaton, Aglay, Josua, Jonas, Calpie, Calphas. appear before me, N.N., in a mild and human form, and do what I desire. (This the conjuror must name.)

The Third Seal

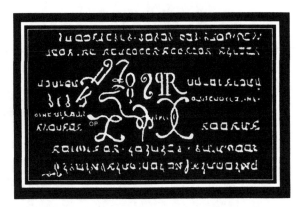

Fig. 4

The ministering Throne Angels of this Seal are the following: Tehom, Haseha, Amarzyom, Schawayt, Chuscha, Zawar, Yahel, La hehor, Adoyahel, Schimuel, Achusaton, Schaddyl, Chamyel, Parymel, Chayo. The special secret of this Throne is that by carrying this Seal with you will cause you to be very agreeable and much beloved, and will also defeat all your enemies.

THE MYSTERY OF THE FOURTH SEAL

Seal of the Ministering Cherubim and Seraphim
with their Characteristics
Conjuration

I, N.N., a servant of God, call upon thee, desire and conjure thee, O spirit Anoch, by the wisdom of Solomon, by the obedience of Isaac, by the blessing of Abraham, by the piety of Jacob and Noe, who did not sin before God, by the serpents of Moses, and by the twelve tribes, and by the most terrible words: Dallia, Dollia, Dollion, Corfuselas, Jazy, Agzy, Ahub, Tilli, Stago, Adoth, Suna, Eoluth, Alos, Jaoth, Dilu, and by all the words through which thou canst be compelled to appear before me in a beautiful, human form, and give what I desire. (This the Conjuror must name.)

The Fourth Seal

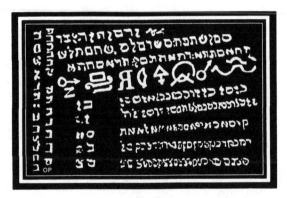

Fig. 5

The most obliging ministering Cherubim and Seraphim of this Seal are the following with their Hebrew calling: Anoch, Sewachar, Chaylon, Esor, Yaron, Oseny, Yagelor, Ehym, Maakyel, Echad, Yalyon, Yagar, Ragat, Ymmat, Chabalym, Schadym.

The special secret of this Seal is that to carry this Seal upon the body will save a person from all misery, and give the greatest fortune and long life.

39

THE MYSTERY OF THE FIFTH SEAL

Seal of the Angels of Power

Conjuration

I, N.N., a servant of God, call upon thee, desire and conjure thee, Spirit Scheol, through the most holy appearance in the flesh of Jesus Christ, by his most holy birth and circumcision, by his sweating of blood in the Garden, by the lashes he bore, by his bitter sufferings and death, by his Resurrection, Ascension and the sending of the Holy Spirit as a comforter, and by the most dreadful words: Dai, Deorum, Ellas, genio Sophiel, Canoel, Elmiach, Richol, Hoamiach, Jerazaol, Vohal, Daniel, Hasios, Tomaiach, Sannul, Damamiach, Sanul, Damabiath, and by those words through which thou canst be conquered, that thou appear before me in a beautiful, human form, and fulfil what I desire. (This the conjuror must name.)

The Fifth Seal

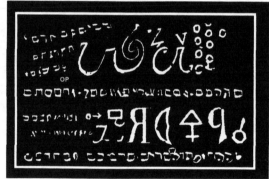

Fig. 6

The most serviceable Angels of Power are the following: Schoel, Hael, Sephiroth, Thamy, Schamayl, Yeehah, Holyl, Yomelo, Hadlam, Mazbaz, Elohaym.

The special secret of this Seal is that if it is laid upon the sick in true faith, it will restore him, if he has not lived the full number of his days. Therefore it is called the Seal of Power.

40

THE MYSTERY OF THE SIXTH SEAL

Seal of the Power Angels seu Potestatum over the Angels and Spirits of All the Elements

Conjuration

I, N.N., a servant of God, desire, call upon and conjure thee, Spirit Alymon, by the most dreadful words, Sather, Ehomo, Geno, Poro, Jehovah, Elohim, Volnah, Denach, Alonlam, Ophiel, Zophiel, Habriel, Eloha, Alesimus, Dileth, Melohim, and by all the holiest words through which thou canst be conquered, that thou appear before me in a mild, beautiful human form, and fulfil what I command thee, so surely as God will come to judge the living and dead. Fiat, Fiat, Fiat.

The Sixth Seal

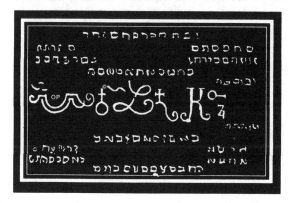

Fig. 7

The most obedient angels of Power, seu Potestates, are the following four elements: Schunmyel, Alymon, Mupiel, Symnay, Semanglaf, Taftyah, Melech, Seolam, Waed, Sezah, Safyn, Kyptip, Taftyarohel, Aeburatiel, Anyam, Bymnam. This is the mystery or Seal of the Might-Angels. The peculiar secret of the Seal is that if a man wears this Seal in bed, he will learn what he desires to know through dreams and visions.

41

THE MYSTERY OF THE SEVENTH SEAL

Seal of the Angels of the Seven Planets and Spirits

Conjuration

I, N.N., a servant of God, call upon, desire, and conjure thee, Ahael, Banech, by the most holy words Agios, Tetragrammaton, Eschiros, Adonai, Alpha and Omega, Raphael, Michael, Uriel, Schmaradiel, Zaday, and by all the known names of Almighty God, by whatsoever thou, Ahael, canst be compelled, that thou appear me in a human form, and fulfil what I desire. Fiat, Fiat, Fiat. (This must be named by the conjuror.)

The Seventh Seal

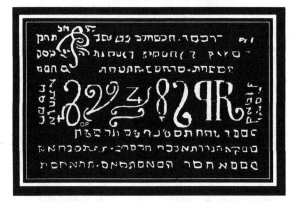

Fig. 8

The most obedient Angels and Spirits of this Seal of the Seven Planets are the following: Ahaeb, Baneh, Yeschnath, Hoschiah, Betodah, Leykof, Yamdus, Zarenar, Sahon. This Seal, when laid upon the treasure earth, or when placed within a mine, will reveal all the precious contents of the mine.

THE

Seventh Book of Moses.

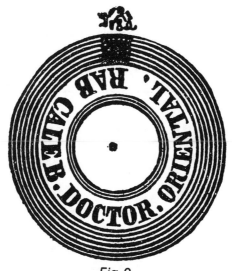

Fig. 9

TRANSLATED BY

RABBI CHALEB.

From the Weimar Bible.

2. The Twelve Tables of the Spirits

EDITOR'S NOTE:

The Twelve Tables of the Spirits are divided into four Tables of the Spirits of the Elements (Air, Fire, Water, and Earth); six Tables of the Planetary Spirits (Saturn, Jupiter, Mars, Sun, Venus, and Mercury); the Eleventh Table of the Spirits, which does not specify the types of spirits invoked; and the Table of the Schemhamforasch, or the 72 Holy Names of God.

Each conjuration is also a translation of the Kabbalistic characters engraved in each Table. This Conjuration is to be said aloud during the magical ceremony of Invocation for each Table.

THE FIRST TABLE OF THE SPIRITS OF THE AIR

Conjuration

Jehovah Father, Deus Adonay Elohe, I cite Thee through Jehovah. Deus Schadday, Eead, I conjure Thee through Adonay.

The First Table

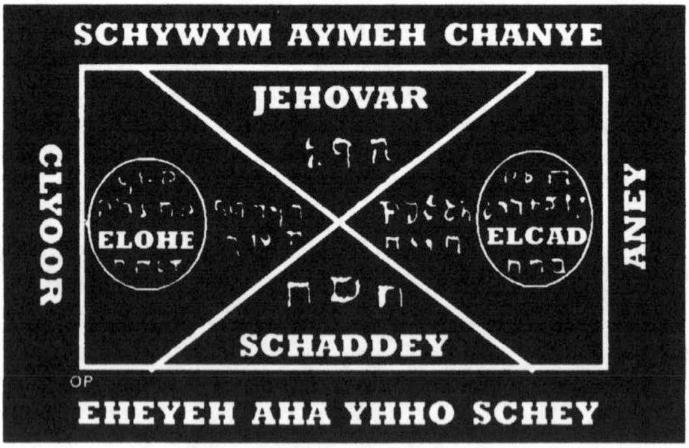

Fig. 10

To carry upon the person the First Table of the Spirits of the Air, who are as quick as thought to help, will relieve the wearer from all necessity.

THE SECOND TABLE OF THE SPIRITS OF FIRE

Conjuration

Aha, I conjure Thee (Tetragrammaton) Aha by Eheye, by Ihros, Eheye,* by Agla Aysch, Jehovah, conjure I Thee, that thou appear unto me.

The Second Table

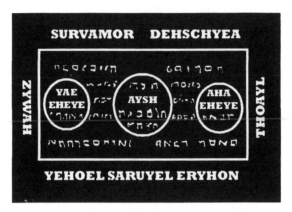

Fig. 11

There is no explanation in the original translation as to what are the uses of this Table.

THE THIRD TABLE OF THE SPIRITS OF WATER

Conjuration

I call upon and command thee Chananya by God Tetragrammaton Eloh. I conjure Thee Yeschaijah by Alpha and Omega, and Thou art compelled through Adonai.

The Third Table

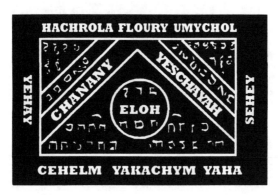

Fig. 12

The Third Table brings great fortune by water, and its spirits will amply supply the treasures of the deep.

THE FOURTH TABLE OF THE SPIRITS OF THE EARTH

Conjuration

I, N.N., command Thee, Awijel, by Otheos as also by Elmez through Agios. I, N.N., a servant of God, conjure Thee, Ahenatos Elijon, as also Adon was cited and called Zebaoth.

The Fourth Table

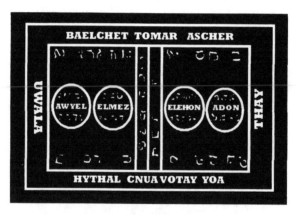

Fig. 13

This Fourth Table will give the treasures of the earth, if it be laid in the earth. Its spirits will give the treasures of the earth at all times.

THE FIFTH TABLE OF SATURN

Conjuration

I, N.N., order, command and conjure Thee Sazlij, by Agios, Sedul, by Sother, Veduij, by Sabaot, Sove, Amonzion* Adoij, by Helohim, Jaho, by the Veritas Jehovah* Kawa, Alha, natos that ye must appear before me in human form, so truly as Daniel overcame and conquered Baal. Fiat, Fiat, Fiat.

The Fifth Table

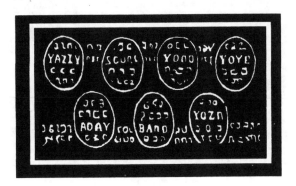

Fig. 14

The Spirits of the Fifth Table of Saturn will serve in everything according to wish. Their Table will bring good luck in play (games of chance).

THE SIXTH TABLE OF JUPITER

Conjuration

I conjure Thee, Spirit Ofel, by Alpha and Omega, Lezo and Yschirios* Ohin Ission* Niva, by Tetragrammaton, Zeno, by Peraclitus* Ohel, by Orlenius, Lima, by Agla*, that ye will obey and appear before me and fulfil my desire, thus in and through the name Elion, which Moses named. Fiat, fiat, fiat.

The Sixth Table

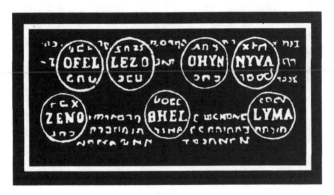

Fig. 15

The Sixth Table of Jupiter assists in overcoming lawsuits, disputes, and in winning at play or games of chance. Their spirits are at all times ready to render assistance.

49

THE SEVENTH TABLE OF MARS

Conjuration

I, N.N., cite Thee, Spirit Emol, by Deus Sachnaton* Luil, by
Acumea* Luiji, by Ambriel*, Tijlaij, by Ehos*, by Jeha, by Zora*
Ageh, by Awoth,* that you appear before me in a beautiful, human
form, and accomplish my desire, thus truly in and through the
anepobeijaron, which Aaron heard and which was prepared for
him. Fiat, fiat, fiat.

The Seventh Table

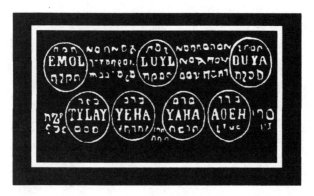

Fig. 16

The Seventh Seal of Mars brings good fortune. In case of
quarrels the Spirits of Mars will help you.

THE EIGHTH TABLE OF THE SUN

Conjuration

I, N.N., conjure Thee, Wrjch by Dalia † Jka, by Doluth*, Auet, by Dilu* Veal, by Anub ✝ Meho, by Igfa* Ymij, by Eloij* that Ye appear before my so true Zebaoth, who was named by Moses, and all the rivers in Egypt were turned into blood.

The Eighth Table

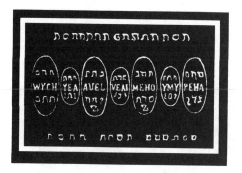

Fig. 17

The Eighth Table of the Spirits of the Sun will help attain honor and wealth, and they also give gold and treasure.

Whenever a cross appears next to a holy name, the conjuror must cross himself. The meaning of the asterisks is not clear.

THE NINTH TABLE OF VENUS

Conjuration

Reta, Kijmah, Yamb, Yheloruvesopijhael, I call upon Thee, Spirit Awel, through God Tetragrammaton, Uhal, by Pomamiach that you will obey my commands and fulfil my desires. Thus truly in and through the name of Esercheije, which Moses named, and upon which followed hail, the like of which was not known since the beginning of the world. Fiat, fiat, fiat.

The Ninth Table

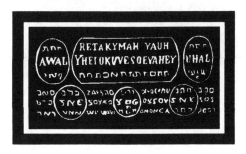

Fig. 18

The Ninth Table of the Spirits of Venus makes one beloved in all respects and makes secrets known through dreams. Its spirits also assist liberally in all kinds of business.

THE TENTH TABLE OF MERCURY

Conjuration

Petasa, Ahor, Havaashar, N.N., cites Thee Spirit Yloij* through God, God Adonaij † Ymah, through God Tetragrammaton † Rawa, through God Emanuel* Ahaij, through Athanatos † that Thou appear before me as truly in and through the name of Adonai, which Moses mentioned, and there appeared grasshoppers. fiat, fiat, fiat.

The Tenth Table

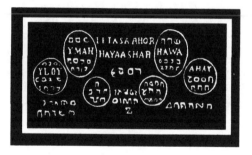

Fig. 19

The Tenth Table of the Spirits of Mercury gives wealth in Chemistry. These spirits contribute treasures of the mines.

Whenever a cross appears next to a holy name, the conjuror must cross himself. The meaning of the asterisks is not clear.

THE ELEVENTH TABLE OF THE SPIRITS

Conjuration

I, N.N., cite Thee, Spirit Yhaij, by El, Yvaij, by Elohim, Ileh, by Elho* Kijlij, by Zebaoth, Taijn Iseij, by Tetragrammaton, Jeha, by Zadaij* Ahel, by Agla that you will obey my orders, as truly in and through the name Schemesumatie, upon which Josua called, and the sun stood still in its course. Fiat, fiat, fiat.

The Eleventh Table

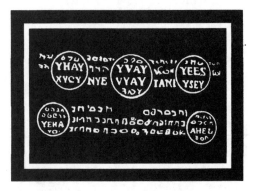

Fig. 20

The Eleventh Table gives good luck and fortune. Its spirits give the treasures of the sea.

THE TWELFTH TABLE OF THE SCHEMHAMFORASCH

(On All Spirits of White and Black Magic)

Conjuration

I, N.N., cite and conjure Thee, Spirit of Schehamforasch, by all the seventy-two holy names of God, that Thou appear before me and fulfil my desire, as truly in and through the name Emanuel, which the three youths Sadrach, Mijsach, and Abednegro sung in the fiery furnace from which they were released. Fiat, fiat, fiat.

The Twelfth Table

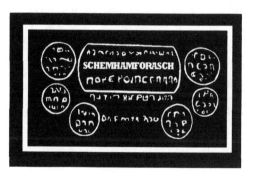

Fig. 21

This Twelfth Table when laid upon the Table or Seal of the Spirits will compel them to appear immediately, and to serve in all things.

THE MINISTERING FORMULAS OR MYSTERIES

The following formulas must be cited by the Twelfth Table during a sun or lunar eclipse:

Astarte, Salomonis familiarum III, Eegum

Spirit of Water, Spirit of Air, Spirit of Earth

Astoreth in Palestina familiari

Schaddaij, Driffon, Agrippa, Magaripp.

Azijelzm, Sinna, familiarum IV, Buch Regum

Schijwin* Aimeh, Chanije, Cijbor

Bealherith ijud Judicum IX, XIII

Adola, Eloheij, Umijchob Channanijah

Adramelech zu Sepharavaijm, Familiaris

Yhaij, Vvaij, Yles, Kijgij

Nisroch, Regis Serucheril Assijris familiaris

Jehuel, Sarwiel, Urikon, Thoijil

Asijma, Virorum Emach familiaris

Barechel, Jomar, Ascher, Uwula

GENERATION SEAL

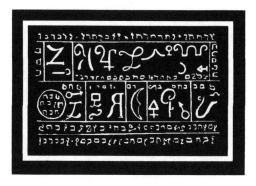

Fig. 22

This Generation Seal, also known as Moloch familiarum or Ammonitarium Ministering Spirits, makes its spirits obedient in all services. At the time of Citation, it must be written on parchment and held in the right hand, but it must not be read.

VOLUME II.

OF THE

SIXTH AND SEVENTH

BOOKS OF MOSES.

FORMULAS

OF THE

MAGICAL KABALA;

OR, THE

MAGICAL ART

OF THE

SIXTH AND SEVENTH BOOKS OF MOSES.

TOGETHER WITH

AN EXTRACT

FROM THE GENUINE AND TRUE

Clavicula of Solomon the King of Israel.

Fig 23

EDITOR'S NOTE:

Volume II gives a collection of seals that were allegedly inscribed on the helmets and breastplates of Moses and Aaron and the Ark of the Covenant, among others. Several formulas, conjurations, citations and dismissions of spirits are also presented, together with their descriptions and their transliterations from Hebrew. The invocations and Hebrew characters used allegedly by Moses to bring about the seven plagues of Egypt are also given in several versions.

In the first version, presented as an "Extract from the Magical Kabala," the transliteration (pronunciation) of the Hebrew characters is given, as well as instructions on how the seals and invocations are to be used. The magician is exhorted to pronounce the "Citation-Formulas" only in the Hebrew language, which is conveniently transliterated for such purposes. The English translations that follow some of the Hebrew pronunciations are for the magician's information only, and are not to be pronounced during the invocations.

In the second version, known as Treatise Sion, are given the seals of the Sixth and the Seventh Books of Moses. The seals of the Sixth Book deal mostly with the Invocations used by Moses to cause the seven plagues of Egypt, as well as the apparition of "The Spirit to Moses on a Burning Bush."

The seals of the Seventh Book deal with the apparition of the Spirit in a Pillar of Fire by night and a Pillar of Clouds by day, the various conjurations and citations of Moses and Eleazar, and the inscriptions on the breastplates and helmets.

The third version, known as Biblia Arcana Magica Alexander, and allegedly published in 1383, deals with the same type of seals as the preceding versions, but the characters within the seals are different. It is to be assumed that these seals correspond to the descriptions and invocations used in the other versions.

The editor has matched the seals in the second version with the descriptions found scattered throughout the original edition in an effort to make the whole intelligible to the reader and magical student.

3. Extract from the Magical Kabala

NOTE:

The Citation-Formulas contained in this book must only be pronounced in the Hebrew language, and in no other. In any other language they have no power whatever, and the Master can never be sure of their effects. For all these words and forms were thus pronounced by the Great Spirit, and have power only in the Hebrew language.

BREASTPLATE OF MOSES

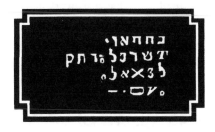

Fig. 24

The Hebrew inscriptions within the seal are pronounced as follows:

JEHOVA, ASER EHEJE CETHER ELEION EHEJE

Their meaning is as follows:

The Most High, whom no eye hath seen, nor tongue spoke; the Spirit which did great acts and performed great wonders. The words of the Breastplate and the Helmet pronounced mean Holiness.

HELMET OF MOSES AND AARON

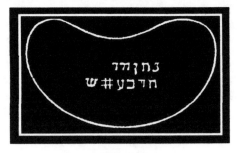

Fig. 25

The Hebrew inscriptions are to be pronounced as follows:

HIEBEL MARE ACTITAS BARNE DONENE ARIAERCH

These are the names which the old Egyptians used instead of the unutterable name of Asser Criel, and are called the "Fire of God," and "Strong Rock of Faith." Whoever wears them on his person will not die a sudden death.

BREASTPLATE OF AARON

Fig. 26

The inscriptions on the seal are to be pronounced as follows:

SADAJAI AMARA ELON HEJIANA VANANEL
PHENATON EBCOEL MERAI

That is, a Prince of Miens, the other leads to Jehova. Through this, God spoke to Moses.

MAGICAL LAW OF MOSES

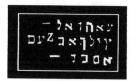

Fig. 27

The inscriptions on the seal are to be read as follows:

AILA HIMEL ADONAIJ AMARA ZEBAOTH CADAS
YESERAIJE HARALIUS

These words are terrible, and will assemble devils or spirits, or they will cause the dead to appear.

THE INSCRIPTION ON THE CHALICE OF HOLINESS

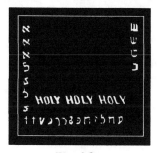

Fig. 28

The inscriptions on the seal are to be read as follows:

ELIAON JOENA EBREEL ELOIJELA AIJEL AGONI SOCHADON

These words are great and mighty. They are names of the Creator and the characters on the Ark of the Covenant.

CONJURATION OF ELEAZAR, THE SON OF AARON

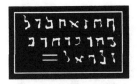

Fig. 29

The inscriptions on the seal are to be read as follows:

UNIEL DILATAN SADAI PANEIM USAMIGRAS CALIPHOS
SASNA SOIM JALAPH

These names, if anyone desires to accomplish anything through the four elements or any other things connected therewith, will prove effective, but they cannot be translated into English.

DISMISSION OF ELEAZAR, THE SON OF AARON

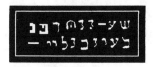

Fig. 30

The inscriptions on the seal are to be read as follows:

LEAY YLI ZIARITE ZELOHABE ET NEGORAMY ZIEN
LATEBM DAMA MECHA RA METI OZIRA

Through this dismission all things dissolve into nothing.

CITATION OF GERMUTHSAI OR LEVIATHAN

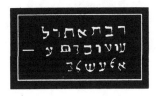

Fig. 31

The inscriptions on the seal are to be read as follows:

LAGUMEN EMANUEL THEREFORI MECHELAG LAIGEL
YAZI ZAZAEL

With these names Eleazar bound and unbound the spirits of the air.

DISMISSION OF LEVIATHAN

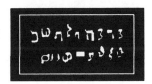

Fig. 32

The inscriptions on the seal are to be read as follows:

MALCOH, SADAIJ, CUBOR DAMABIAH MENKIE
LEJABEL MANIAH IJEJAVAI

That is, Strong, Might spirit of hell, go back into thine own works, in the name of Jehova.

BALAAM'S SORCERY

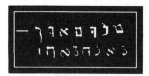

Fig. 33

The inscriptions on this seal are to be read as follows:

MELOCH, HEL ALOKIM TIPHRET HOD JESATH

This brings vengeance upon enemies, and must not be disregarded because it contains the names of the Seven Tables of the Covenant.

EGYPT

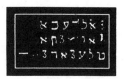

Fig. 34

The inscriptions on the seal are to be read as follows:

TANABTIAN AINATEN PAGNIJ AIJOLO ASNIA HICHAIFALE
MATAE HABONR HIJCERO

With these words Moses spake to the sorcerers in Egypt. They signify: "The Lord appeared to his servant in the fire, to seal the earth in its four quarters, and the nether earth."

CONJURATION OF THE LAWS OF MOSES

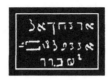

Fig. 35

The inscription on the seal must be read as follows;

AIJCON DUNSANAS PETHANIR THRIJGNIR IJON
CIJNA NATER LAVIS PISTOIN

If you wish to pronounce these words you must fast for three days, and you can perform wonders therewith. They cannot be translated on account of the Hebrew characters.

GENERAL CITATION OF MOSES ON ALL SPIRITS

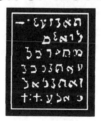

Fig. 36

The inscriptions on the seal are to be read as follows:

ELION GOEUA ADONAIJ CADAS EBREEL, ELOIL ELA AGIEL, AIJONI SACHADON, ESSUSELAS ELOHIM, DELIION JAU ELIJULA, DELIA JARI ZAZAEL PALIEMAO UMIEL, ONALA DILATUM SADATJ, ALMA JOD JAEL THAMA

This citation is great and mighty. They are the names of the Creator, and the names of the two Cherubim on the Mercy Seat, Zarall and Jael.

67

DISMISSION OF MOSES

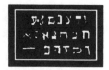

Fig. 37

The inscriptions on this seal are to be read as follows:

WASZEDIM BACHANDA HEZANHAD JEHOV ELOHIM ASSER
EHOIE ZALIM

GENERAL CITATION OF MOSES ON ALL SPIRITS

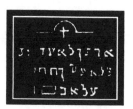

Fig. 38

The inscriptions on the seal are to be read as follows:

AHEZERAIJE COMITEJON SEDE LEJI THOMOS SASMAGATA
BIJ UL IJCOS JOUA ELOIJ ZAWAIJM

These are the high and powerful utterances that Moses employed in the awakening of the Leviathan, in order to compel him to serve his Lord. The first cannot be uttered and was used by the first inhabitants of earth as a mighty lord. The whole is good, but not everyone can obtain it in perfection without severe discipline.

CHARACTERS ON THE LEFT SIDE OF THE ARK OF THE COVENANT OF THE MOST HIGH

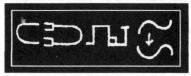

Fig. 39

CHARACTERS ON THE RIGHT SIDE OF THE ARK OF THE COVENANT OF THE MOST HIGH

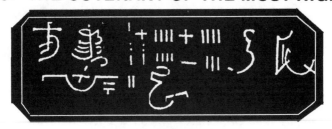

Fig. 40

Hear, Oh Israel, the Lord our God is God alone.

CONJURED SPIRIT APPEARS ON A PILLAR OF FIRE

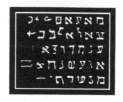

Fig. 41

The inscriptions on the seal are to be said as follows:

AFFABIJ ZIEN, JERAMIJE LATABI DAMAJESANO NOIJ LIJOIJ LEAIJ GLIJ EIJLOIJ LIECLE LOATE ELI ELI MECHARAMETHIJ RIJBISAS SA FU AZIRA REACHA

The Citation names the twelve evil spirits of man, through the help of the Father, of the Hebrew Eli. It is terrible.

CONJURED SPIRIT APPEARS ON A PILLAR OF CLOUDS

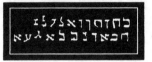 Fig. 42

The inscriptions on the seal are to be read as follows:

KAHAI CONOR ANUHEC ZELOHAE ZOLE HEBEI EDE NEGO RANEIJ HAHABE GIZAON

Appendix to the General Citation of Moses on All Spirits

We, N.N., in this circle, conjure and cite this spirit Fatenovenia, with all his adherents, to appear here in this spot, to fulfil our desires, in the name of the three holy angels, Schomajen Sheziem, Roknion Averam, Kandile, Brachat Chaijdalic, Ladabas, Labul, Raragil, Bencul, in the name of God. Amen.

THREE NEW SIGNS WITH FROGS, LICE AND PESTILENCE

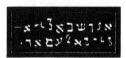 Fig. 43

The inscriptions on the seal to be read as follows:

ABLAN, AGEISTAN, ZORATAN JURAN, NONDIERAS PORTAEPHIAS POGNIJ AIZAMAI

THREE NEW SIGNS WITH CATTLE, PESTILENCE BLACK SMALLPOX AND HAIL

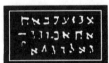 Fig. 44

The inscriptions on the seal are to be read as follows:
ARARITA ZAIJN THANAIN, MIORATO RAEPI SATHONIK PETHANIT CASTAS LUCAS CALBERA NATUR SIGAIM

SIGNS OF GRASSHOPPERS AND DARKNESS

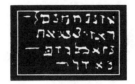

Fig. 45

The inscriptions on the seal are to be said as follows:

HASSADAY HAYLOES, LUCASIM ELAYH JACIHAGA,
YOININO, SEPACTICAS BARNE LUD CASTY:

THE SPIRIT APPEARS IN THE BURNING BUSH

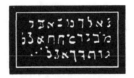

Fig. 46

The inscriptions on the seal are to be read as follows:

BABA CUCI HIEBU ZIADHI ELENEHET NA VEAN VIE
ACHYA SALNA

The spirit which appears here is God himself.

MOSES CHANGES THE STAFF INTO A SERPENT

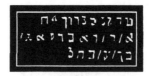

Fig. 47

The inscriptions on the seal are to be read as follows:

MICRATA RAEPI SATHONIK PETHANISCH, PISTAN IJTTINGE HIJGATIGN IJGHUZIAN TEMGARONUSNIA CASTAS LACIAS ASTAS IJECON CIJNA CALTERA CAPHAS

MOSES CHANGES WATER INTO BLOOD

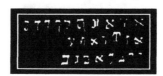

Fig. 48

The inscriptions on the seal are to be read as follows:

ABEN AGLA MANDEL SLOP SIEHAS MALIM HAJATH HAJADOSCH IJONEM, CEDAS EBREEL AMPHIA, DEMISRAEL MUELLE LEAGIJNS AMANIHA

EXTRACT FROM THE TRUE CLAVICULA OF SOLOMON AND THE GIRDLE OF AARON

This was bequeathed as a testament to all the wise magicians, which all the old Fathers possessed and employed, to have and fulfill all things through the illustrious power of the mighty God Jehovah, as He, the great Monarch, gave to His creatures, who worship Him day and night with reverence and fear, who call loudly upon His name in secret, and sigh to Him as their origin, as of Him and from Him existing reasonable beings, as on the point of being involved with the pains of the elements, who strive after the highest being to and with God. To these He has given this, who will not forget Him in the pleasures of this world, who, still bearing suffering without forgetting the reality, nor the perishing lustre of the world.

PRINCIPAL CITATION ON ALL MINISTERING SPIRITS OF THE AIR AND OF EARTH, THE LIKE OF WHICH MANASSES AND SOLOMON USED AS THE TRUE KEY SOLOMONIS REGIS ISRAEL

You must stand on a prominent rock, hold a palm twig in your right hand, and wear a wreath of laurel around the temples. Then turn toward the east and say:

ALIJA LAIJA LAUMIN OTHEON!

At this time, a halo of light will surround you, and when you become aware of this light, fall upon your knees and worship. Then say in an audible voice the words inscribed in the following seal. You must speak slowly and distinctly.

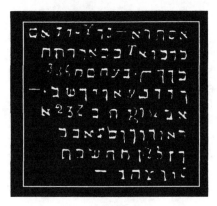

Fig. 49

ELIAM YOENA ADONAI CADUS EBREEL ELOYELA AGIEL, AYOM
SACHADON OSSUSELAS ELOYM DE LIOMAR ELYNLA LELIA
YAZI ZAZALL UNNEL OVELA DILATAM SADAY ALMA PANAIM
ALYM CANAL DENSY USAMI YASAS CALIPI CALFAS SASNA
SAFFA SADOJA AGLATA PANTOMEL AMRIEL AZIEN PHANATON
SARZE PENERION YA EMANUEL JOD JALAPH AMPHIA THAN
DOMIRAEL ALOWIN.

CHARACTERS

CHARACTERS.

B A m n lazies ala phonfin agaloyes pyol paerteon theserym.

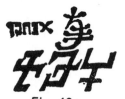

basimel Jael barionia.

apiolet cenet.

Fig. 49a

B A M N LAZIES ALA PHONFIN AGALOYES PYOL PAERTEON

THESERYM. BASIMEL JAEL BARIONIA

APIOLET CENET.

BIBLIA,

ARCANA MAGICA ALEXANDER,

ACCORDING TO THE

Tradition of the Sixth and Seventh Books of Moses,

BESIDES

MAGICAL LAWS.

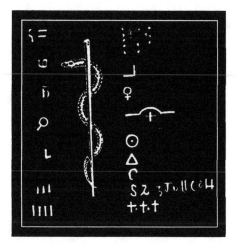

Ex Verbis Revelatis (II) Intellectui Sigillati
Verbis.

NUNC APOSTOLICA ✠ CONSECRATIONE

DE NOVO CONFIRMATO.

Script. de Ellbio.

ANNO MCCCLXXXIII.

Fig.49b

III.

EXTRACT

FROM THE

MAGICAL KABALA,

OF THE

SIXTH AND SEVENTH

BOOKS OF MOSES.

BY

S. T. N.

Translated for the first time from the Cuthan-Samaritan Language into English.

———

ANNO MDCCXXVI.

TRANSLATOR'S PREFACE.

SINCE the Oriental transcript of this work was imperfect in many parts, the translation of it had to be taken according to the great original book, on account of the purity of its text, and, therefore, it won for itself the advantage of understanding and completing the exercises with serenity and confidence. The translator, in the meantime believes, that no one, who feels honestly called to these things, can ever be made the subject of ill-fortune, or be deceived by the wiles and deceptions of the old serpent, the inevitable fate that will and must fall to his lot under any other exorcisms, and that he may cheerfully and safely move thence, because only the angels of God will perform the service required by Him.

Fig. 49c

4. Treatise Sion

EDITOR'S NOTE:

Treatise Sion is the second version of the seals described in the preceding version known as an "Extract from the Magical Kabala." Treatise Sion is divided into the Treatise of the Sixth Book of Moses and the Treatise of the Seventh book of Moses. The Treatise is alternately known as the Revelation of Zion. Each seal and its descriptions are given as chapters of each book.

INTRODUCTION AND BEGINNING

The Vestibule of Entrance

The language and manuscript of this rare and eternal monument of light, and of a higher wisdom, are borrowed from the Cuthans, a tribe of the Samaritans, who were called Cuthim in the Chaldee dialect according to the Talmud, and they were so called in a spirit of derision. They were termed sorcerers because they taught in Cutha, their original place of abode, and afterward in Samaria, the Kabala or Higher Magic (Book of Kings). Caspar, Melchior and Balthazar, the chosen archpriests, are shining lights among the Eastern magicians. They were kings and teachers — the first priest/teachers of this glorious knowledge — and from these Samaritans-Cuthans, who were called Nergal according to the traditions of the Talmud, originated the Gypsies, who, through degeneracy, lost the consecration of their primordial powers.

EDITOR's NOTE:

The following Laws of Entrance are reproduced, unedited, as they were given in the original edition. For the most part they are instructions on the magician's preparations prior to and during the ritual. Some editorial comments follow some of the most abstruse instructions.

LAWS OF ENTRANCE

1. Before you can enter the temple of consecrated light, you must purify your soul and body during thirteen days. (**Editor:** Purification can be accomplished by abstinence from sex, meat and drugs, including alcohol and tobacco. Moderate fasting is advised by many magicians during this period.)

2. As a brother and disciple of the new covenant, or as a Christian, you must receive the Holy Sacrament for the glorification of the three kings — Caspar, Melchior and Balthasar.

3. Three holy masses must be read as often as you make use of this book in your priestly service with your intention fixed upon the three glorified kings.

4. You must provide yourself with a ram's horn, wherewith to call together the angels and spirits. This horn must be included in your intentions of the holy mass.

5. You must wear a breastplate of parchment, ten inches high and ten inches wide, inscribed with the names of the twelve apostles with the five-fold name of Schemhamforasch, in the same order that it is placed on the last leaf.
(**Editor:** See Fig. 50.)

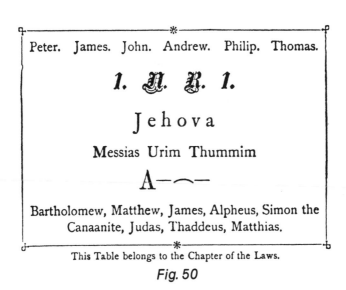

Fig. 50

6. You must draw a circle around you upon white paper, or upon sky blue silk. Its circumference shall be thirteen feet, and at the distance of each foot, one of the following names must be written: Moseh, Messias, Aaron, Jehova, Adoni, Jesus, Christus, Caspar, Melchior, Balthasar. Al. Al. Al.

7. Between each name you must place the holy symbol of Horet: ——†— —†—— or —†—— ——†—.

8. The breastplate must be included in the intention of the holy mass.

9. Through consecration with holy three king's water and with three burning wax tapers, you must finally pronounce a benediction over this book, the horn, the breastplate, and the circle, after reading a well-selected mysterious ritual. (**Editor:** For those would-be magicians who cannot get holy three king's water, they can substitute that substance with holy water or salt water, salt being a highly purifying mineral. The "well-selected, mysterious ritual" can be any appropriate ritual from any of the grimoires, such as the Clavicle of Solomon.)

10. You may enter alone, or begin this great work with two companions, by day or night, but always from the first to the thirteenth of the month, and during the thirteenth day, and through the whole night of the new moon, and also during the full moon, when thje three planets, Saturn, Mars and Jupiter, are visible in the heavens on the day of exorcism, either singly or together.

11. You must always stand with your face toward Zion, or toward the rising of the sun.

12. He who refuses a copy of this book, or who suppresses it or steals it, will be seized with eternal trembling like Cain, and the angels of god will depart from him.

TREATISE OF THE SIXTH BOOK OF MOSES

CHAPTER I. THE SPIRIT APPEARS UNTO MOSES IN A BURNING BUSH

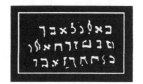

Fig. 50a

Conjuration

KALUKU! UBESU! LAWISU! — Arise and teach me.
Calls with voice and horn as instructed.

CHAPTER II. MOSES CHANGES THE STAFF INTO A SERPENT

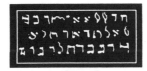

Fig. 51

Conjuration

TUWISU! KAWISU! LAWISU! - Arise and change this staff into a serpent.

Calls with voice and horn as instructed.

CHAPTER III. MOSES CHANGES WATER INTO BLOOD

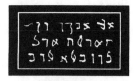

Fig. 52

AKAUATIU! TUWALU! LABATU! — Arise and change this water into blood.

Calls with voice and horn as instructed.

CHAPTER IV. THREE NEW SIGNS WITH FROGS, MICE, LICE AND SIMILAR VERMIN

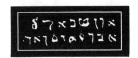

Fig. 53

Conjuration

ADUS! BAACHUR! ARBU! ULU! — Frogs, mice, lice and similar vermin arise in our service.

CHAPTER V. THREE SIGNS OF CATTLE PESTILENCE, BLACK SMALL POX AND HAIL

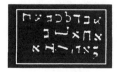

Fig. 54

Conjuration

ABULL, BAA! — Pestilence, black smallpox and hail, arise in our service.

CHAPTER VI. THREE SIGNS WITH GRASSHOPPERS AND DARKNESS

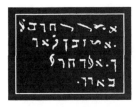

Fig. 55

Conjuration

ARDUSI! DALUSI! — Grasshoppers, darkness, arise in our service.

These are the plagues which the Cuthians often employed in their exorcisms for punishment.

CHAPTER VII. GENERAL CITATION OF MOSES ON ALL SPIRITS

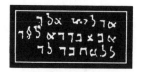

Fig. 56

Conjuration

ADULAL! ABULAL! LEBUSI! — Arise and bring before me the spirit N. (Spirit's name must be uttered.)

Calls with voice and horn as instructed.

THE PENTAGON OR OMNIPOTENT FIVE CORNERS

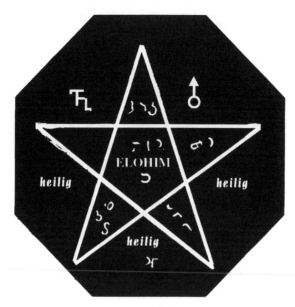

Fig. 56a

This mysterious figure must be written before the conjuration, in the open air and on the ground, with consecrated chalk or with the index finger of the right hand dipped in holy three-king's water, the same as it is written on the illustration, but each line must be thirteen feet in length. The conjuror then kneels in the center of the star, facing east with head uncovered, and calls out thirteen times, with great faith and fervor, the names of the three kings, Caspar, Melchior and Balthasar. He then calls out, with equal sentiment, the most sacred name of Elohim, 375 times. This conjuration can only take place during the first three days or nights of the new or full moon, or when Saturn, Mars and Jupiter are visible in the heavens, as established in the Laws of Entrance.

TREATISE OF THE SEVENTH BOOK OF MOSES

CHAPTER I. THE SPIRIT APPEARS IN A PILLAR OF FIRE BY NIGHT

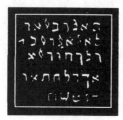

Fig. 57

Conjuration

TALUBSI! LATUBUSI! KALUBUSI! ALUSI! — Arise and bring me the pillar of Fire that I may see.

The name of each angel must be called out three times to the four quarters of the earth, first with the voice, then with the horn.

CHAPTER II. THE SPIRIT APPEARS IN A PILLAR OF CLOUD BY DAY

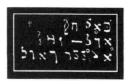

Fig. 58

Conjuration

BUAL! COME! AUL! ARISE! TUBO! COME! WEGULO! ARISE!

The blowing of the horn must be repeated.

CHAPTER III. BALAAM'S SORCERY

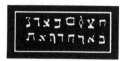

Fig. 59

Conjuration

ONU, BASCHBA, NISCHOAZ HUERETZ — In the name of God I conjure the earth.

CHAPTER IV. EGYPT

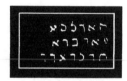

Fig. 60

Conjuration of Three Angels

GEBRIL! MEACHUEL! NESANEL! — By the lamp of the threefold eternal light, let N.N. (name of spirit) appear before me.

Three calls with the voice and three with the horn.

CHAPTER V. CONJURATION OF THE LAWS OF MOSES

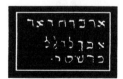

Fig. 61

KEISEHU, NISCHBA, LAWEMSO — How to be God, so swarest Thou to our parents.

Prayer

Eternal of Eternals! Jehovah of Light, Adonai of Truth! Messiah of the All Merciful! Jesus Christ the Beloved and All Redemption and Love! Thou hast said: Who seeth me seeth also the Father. Father, eternal Father of the old and new convenants. Triune Father, Triune Son, Triune Spirit, our Father, I beseech and conjure Thee by the eternal words of Thy eternal truth.

Now read the 17th chapter of John or Jesus' prayer.

Closing Prayer of the Conjuration of the Law

Eternal God Jehovah, Thou hast said: Ask and it shall be given you. I pray that Thou mayest hear Thy servants Caspar, Melchior and Balthasar, the archpriest of Thy fountain of light! I pray that thou mayest bid thine angels to purify me from all sin; that they may breathe upon me in love, and that they may cover me with the shadow of their wings. Send them down! This is my prayer in peace!

CHAPTER VI. GENERAL CITATION OF MOSES ON ALL SPIRITS

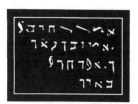

Fig. 62

There is no conjuration or description accompanying this figure.

*CHAPTER VII. GENERAL CITATION OF MOSES ON ALL SPIRITS

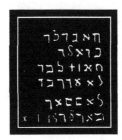

Fig. 63

Conjuration

TUBATLU! BUALU! TULATU! LABUS! UBLISI! — Let there appear and bring before me the spirit of N.N. (name of spirit).

Each of these five omnipotent angels must be called three times toward the four quarters of the world, first with the voice then with the horn, to make a total of six calls.

DISMISSAL OF MOSES

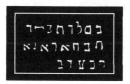

Fig. 64

Conjuration

UBELUTUSI! KADUKULITI! KEBUTZI! — Take away from my presence the spirit of N.N.

Twelve calls with the voice and twelve calls with the horn for each name.

*CHAPTER VII. CONJURATION OF ELEAZAR

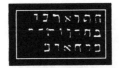

Fig. 65

DUWATU, BUWATIE, BEMAIM - I come to you on the water! Bring me up N.N.! (name of spirit)

*EDITOR'S NOTE: In the original book there are two Chapters VII, which could have been an error on the part of the author. I have decided not to change them.

DISMISSAL OF ELEAZAR

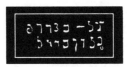

Fig. 66

Conjuration

ORUM, BOLECTN, UBAJOM — Cursed by night and by day!

CHAPTER VIII. CITATION OF QUERNITHAY OR LEVIATHAN

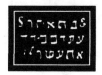

Fig. 67

Conjuration

ELUBATEL, EBUHUEL, ATUESUEL!

Each name must be repeated three times. These, as well as the following invocations, contain only the peculiar names of the angels of omnipotence who will permit the conjured spirits to appear, or will compel them to appear by force.

DISMISSAL

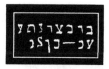

Fig. 68

Conjuration

I beseech thee, angel Elubatel, conduct N.N. (name of spirit) from my presence.

Each angel's name must be pronounced three times with the voice and three times the horn must be blown, each time towards the four quarters of the earth.

CHAPTER IX. MAGICAL LAWS OF MOSES

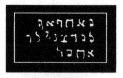

Fig. 69

Conjuration

KUTA-AL, LEWUWAT — We are great! Our Hearts!

Prayer

Oh Lord, arise, that my enemies may be destroyed and that they may fly; that those who hate Thee may be scattered like smoke — drive them away. As wax melteth before the fire, so pass away all evil doers before God, for God has given thee the kingdom. Pour out Thy wrath over them. Thy wrath seize them. Thou shalt stand upon leopards and adders, and Thou shalt subdue the lion and dragon. With God only can we do great things. He will bring them under our feet.

CHAPTER X. HELMET OF MOSES AND AARON

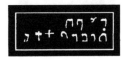

Fig 70

WOCHUTU, TUKAL, BESCHUFA, GUTAL — If I shall sin, I shall blow with the great horn.

Here the horn must be blown three times towards the four quarters of the earth. For the ram's horn, in the old covenant, is the symbol of omnipotence and of purification, or of beauty, truth and holiness.

CHAPTER XI. BREASTPLATE OF MOSES

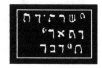

Fig. 71

Conjuration

SCHEDUSI, WEDUSE, TIWISI. — I have sinned, I shall sin.

Prayer

Eternal God of our All! Our god! Hear our voice, spare and have mercy upon us. Accept our prayer in mercy and with pleasure. I have sinned. I have committed transgressions. I have sinned before Thee. I have done that which is displeasing unto Thee here in the earth. For the sake of Thy great name pardon me all the sins and iniquities and transgressions which I have committed against Thee from my youth. Perfect again all the holy names which I have blemished, Great Champion, terrible, highest God, eternal Lord, God Sabaoth.

CHAPTER XII. BREASTPLATE OF AARON

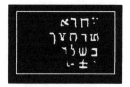

Fig. 72

Conjuration

DEHUTU, EUWSALTU, BESCHOLAM — You have sinned. I shall sin in peace.

Prayer

The Lord, King of all Kings, holy and praised is He, the Father, God, Son of God, the Holy Spirit of God are three in one among these three. In the power of Thy might and Thy right, release those that are bound, receive the prayer of thy people, strengthen us, purify us, Oh terrible Hero, us who worship Thine name. Protect them as the apple of Thine eye, bless them, cleanse them, repay them always in mercy and justice. Mighty, Holy Lord, reward Thy congregration with Thy great goodness. Thou, the only and exalted God, appear unto thy people with Thy holy name; receive and remember our prayer; hearken unto our cries, Thou who knowest all secrets and who knowest our desire.

Here the horn must be blown as previously instructed.

CHAPTER XIII. THE CHALICE OF HOLINESS

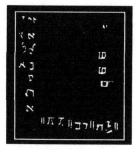

Fig. 73

Conjuration

Al, Al, Al — Arise, Thou eternal Angel!

This must be repeated three times in a loud voice, and the horn must also be blown three times, for he is an angel of the sanctuary.

Prayer

Thou that art, wast, and wilt be in the old and new covenant! Eternal, Jehovah, Jesus Christ, Messias, All Beautiful, All True, All Holy! All Loving and All Merciful in the old and in the new covenant. Thou hast said: Heaven and earth shall pass away, but my words shall not pass away. Thou hast said: I came not to destroy the old covenant, but to fulfill it. Thou hast said: He who sees me, sees the Father. Thou hast said: If ye have true faith, ye can perform the wonders which I have done, yea, ye will perform yet much greater wonders than I have done. Come also to me for the sake of my faith, come also unto me for the sake of Moses, Thy messenger of faith. Reveal also to me Thy mysterious name from Jehovah, as Thou once did to Thy fire prophet Moses in solitude. Come, and say unto me in love, through the heart of Moses and with the tongue of Aaron: SCAHEBUAL! I shall come!

FOR THE LEFT HAND

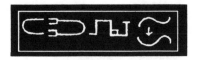

Fig. 74

These signs were used at the time of burnt offerings in the holy temple.

FOR THE RIGHT HAND

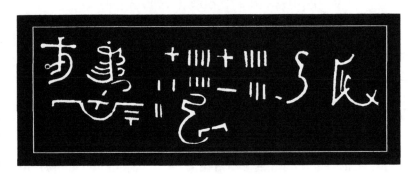

Fig. 75

These are also symbolical of the plagues of Pharoah in Egypt. SCHEMA ISRAEL ADONAI ELOHJEINU, ADONAI ECHAD. — Hear, O Israel, the Lord our God, the Lord is one.

BIBLIA

Arcana Magica Alexandri (Magi),

ACCORDING TO

(REVEALED) TRADITION OF THE SIXTH AND SEVENTH

BOOKS OF MOSES.

TOGETHER WITH THE

MAGICAL LAWS.

Ex Verbis H. (human) Intellectui Sigillatis Verbis.

Nunc Apostoli— ✠ (Anctoritate) Consecrata de Novo Confirmata
✠ ✠ ✠ (Licentia.)

Script de Eppbio.

_____

ANNO MCCCXXXVIII.

Biblia Arcana Magica Alexander,

ACCORDING TO THE TRADITION OF THE

SIXTH AND SEVENTH BOOKS OF MOSES.

TOGETHER WITH THE MAGICAL LAWS.

Ex Verbis (H) Intellectui Sigillatis Verbis Nunc Apostolica ✠

Consecrat de Nove Confirmati ✠ ✠

SCRIPT DE ELSTRO.

MCCCLXXXIII.

Fig. 75a

97

5. Biblia Arcana Magica Alexander

TRADITION OF THE SIXTH BOOK OF MOSES

CHAPTER I. THE SPIRIT APPEARS IN A BURNING BUSH

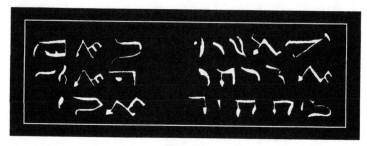

Fig. 76

CHAPTER II. MOSES CHANGES THE STAFF INTO A SERPENT

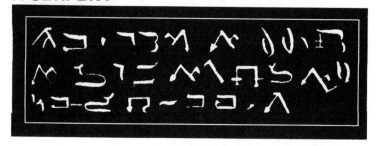

Fig. 77

CHAPTER III. MOSES CHANGES WATER INTO BLOOD

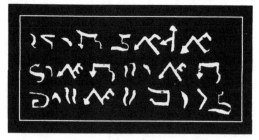

Fig. 78

CHAPTER IV. THREE NEW SIGNS WITH FROGS, LICE AND SIMILAR VERMIN

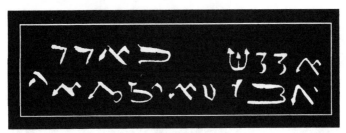

Fig. 79

CHAPTER V. THREE SIGNS OF CATTLE PESTILENCE BLACK SMALLPOX AND HAIL

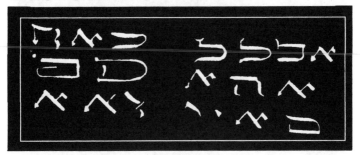

Fig. 80

CHAPTER VI. THREE SIGNS WITH GRASS-HOPPERS AND LOCUSTS

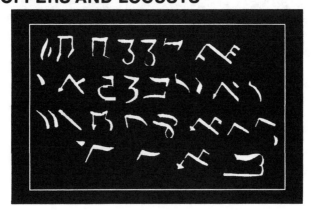

Fig. 81

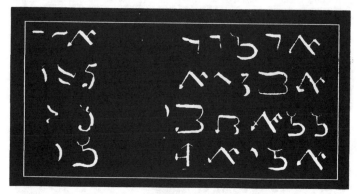

Fig. 82

THE PENTAGON

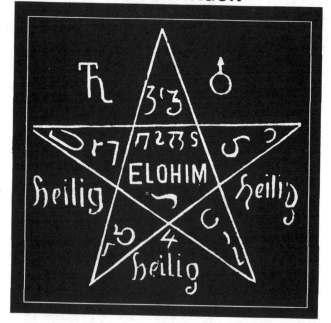

Fig. 83

TRADITION OF THE SEVENTH BOOK OF MOSES

CHAPTER I. THE SPIRIT APPEARS IN A PILLAR OF FIRE BY NIGHT

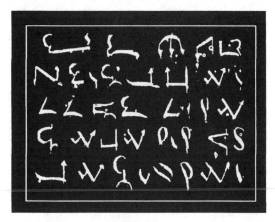

Fig. 84

CHAPTER II. THE SPIRIT APPEARS IN A PILLAR OF CLOUD BY DAY

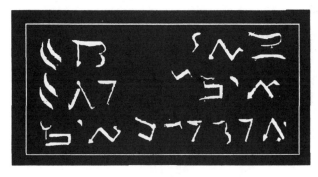

Fig. 85

CHAPTER III. BALAAM'S SORCERY

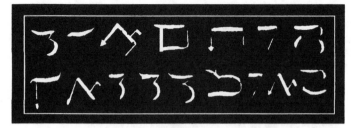

Fig. 86

CHAPTER IV. EGYPT

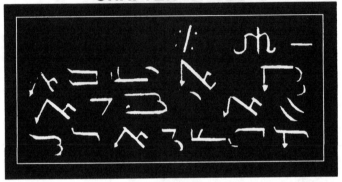

Fig. 87

CHAPTER V. CONJURATION OF THE LAWS OF MOSES

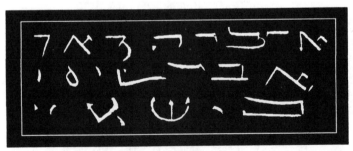

Fig. 88

CHAPTER VI. GENERAL CITATION OF ALL SPIRITS

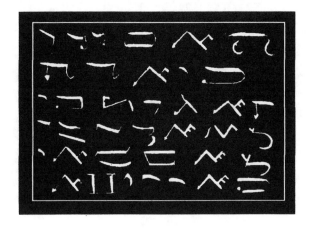

Fig. 89

DISMISSAL OF MOSES

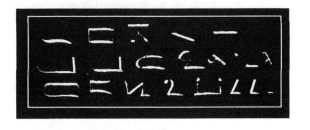

Fig. 90

MAGICAL LAWS OF MOSES

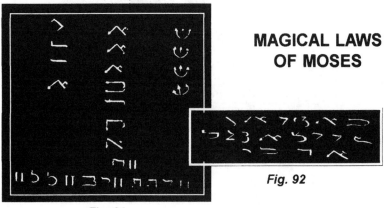

Fig. 92

Fig. 91

BREASTPLATE OF MOSES

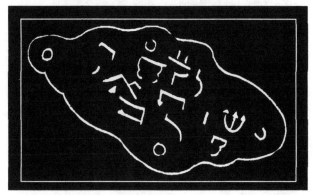

Fig. 93

HELMET OF MOSES AND AARON

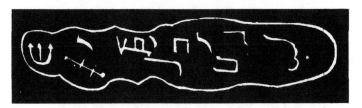

Fig. 94

BREASTPLATE OF AARON

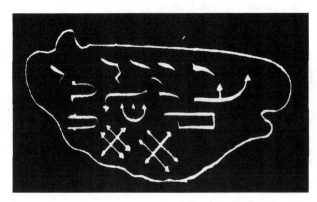

Fig. 95

FOR THE LEFT HAND

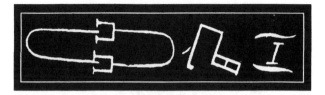

Fig. 96

FOR THE RIGHT HAND

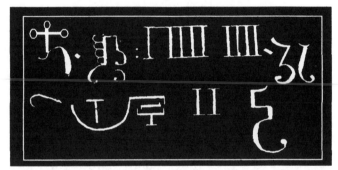

Hear, oh Israel, the Lord our God is God alone. Amen   *Fig. 97*

CONJURATION OF ELEAZAR

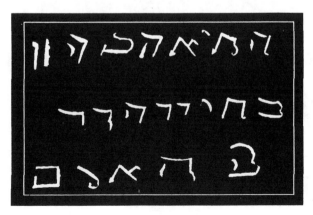

Fig. 98

DISMISSAL OF ELEAZAR

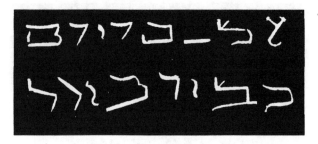

Fig. 99

CITATION OF QUERMILLAM OR LEVIATHAN

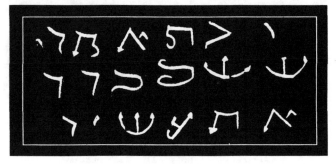

Fig. 100

DISMISSAL OF QUERMILLAM OR LEVIATHAN

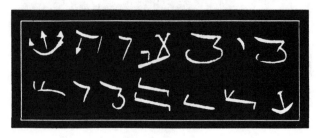

Fig. 98

6. APPENDIX

Magical (Spirit Commado) beside the Black Raven

Romae ad Arcanum Pontificatus under Pope Alexander VI

Printed in 1501 AD

Instructions

If you want to compel spirits to appear visibly before you and render you obedience, observe the following instructions:

1. Keep God's commandments as much as possible.

2. Build and trust solely upon the might and power of God: believe firmly in his omnipotent help in your work, and the spirits will become your servants and will obey you.

3. Continue your citations and do not cease, even if the spirits do not appear at once. Be steadfast in your work and have faith, for the doubter will obtain nothing.

4. Take special note of the times for the invocation:

Monday night - from eleven until three.
Tuesday night - from ten until two
Wednesday night - from twelve until three
Thursday night - from twelve until two
Friday night - from ten until three
Saturday night - from ten until twelve
Sunday Sabbath keep holy unto the Lord Sabaoth, Adonai, Tetragrammaton

5. The time must be the new moon, that is, the moon must be waxing.

6. Trace the circle on Figure 102 on parchment with the blood of young white doves. The size of the circle is optional.

7. The circle must be consecrated before the ceremony, with the following words:

Ego (name of the conjuror), consecro et benedico istum circulum per Nomina Dei Attisimi in ec Scripta, ut sit mihi et omnibus Scutum et Protectio dei Fortissimi Elohim Invincibilie contra omnes malignos Spiritus, gerurmque Potestates. In Nomine Dei Patris Dei Filii Dei Spiritus Sancti. Amen.

Upon your entrance into this circle, speak as follows: Tetragrammaton, Theos, Ischiros, Athanatos, Messias, Imas, Kyrie Eleison. Amen.

After you have entered the circle, begin your operation with the following prayer from the Ninety-first psalm:

He that dwelleth in the secret place of the Most High shall abide under the shadow of the Almighty. I will say of the Lord, He is my refuge and my fortress, my God, in Him will I trust. Surely He shall deliver me from the snare of the fowler and from the noisome pestilence. He shall cover thee with His feathers and under his wings shalt thou trust. His truth shall be thy shield and thy buckler. Thou shalt not be afraid of the terror by night nor of the arrow that flieth by day. Because thou hast made the Lord, which is my refuge, even the Most High, thy habitation. There shall no evil befall thee, neither shall any plague come nigh thy dwelling. Because he has set his love upon me, therefore will I deliver him. I will set him on high because he has known my name. He will call upon me and I will answer him. I will be with him in trouble. I will deliver him and honor him. With long life will I satisfy him and show him My salvation. Even so help me and all them that seek thy holy God the Father + God the Son + God the Holy Ghost +, Amen.

CIRCLE WRITTEN ON PARCHMENT

with the

BLOOD OF WHITE YOUNG DOVES

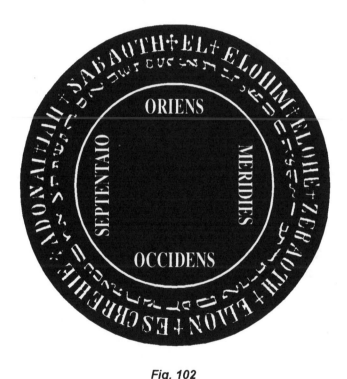

Fig. 102

7. Citation of the Seven Great Princes

EDITOR'S NOTE:

The names of the seven great princes are Aziel, Marbuel, Mephistophilis, Barbuel, Aziabel and Anituel. In their seals their names have been Latin-ized and for that reason they all terminate in "is." For example, Arielis, Barbuelis, and so on.

REMARKS

Following is some information regarding the appearances and provinces of the various spirits.

AZIEL — is a very prompt treasure spirit of the earth and of the sea. He appears in the form of a wild ox.

ARIEL — is a very serviceable spirit, and appears in the form of a ferocious dog. He commands the lost treasures of the land and sea.

MARBUEL — appears in the form of an old lion. He delivers the treasures of the water and of the land, and assists in obtaining all secret knowledge and honors.

MEPHISTOPHILIS — is ready to serve, and appears in the form of a youth. He is willing to serve in all skilled arts, and gives the spiritus Servos, otherwise called "familiars." He brings treasures from the earth and from the deep very quickly.

BARBUEL — is a master of all arts and all secret knowledge, a great master of all treasure. He is very accomodating, and appears with alacrity in the form of a wild hog.

AZIABEL — is a prince of the water and mountain spirits and their treasures. He is amiable and wears a large pearl crown.

ANITUEL — appears in the form of a serpent of paradise. He confers great wealth and honors according to wish.

Instructions

The seals or General Characters of the Seven Great Princes must be written upon virgin parchment with the blood of butterflies, at the time of the full moon. The Seven Great Princes have among them some of the legions of crown-spirits who were expelled from Heaven, according to tradition.

Mundus ater cum illis
Me pactum dicit habere
Sed me teque Deus
Te illo custodiat omnes.

CITATIONS AND SEALS

Citation of AZIEL

✠   ✠   ✠

AZIELIS

Seal or Character for Coercion and Obedience.

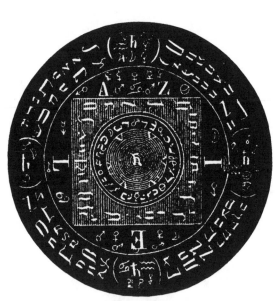

Fig. 103

Agla, Cadelo, Samba, Caclem, Awenhatoacoro, Aziel, Zorwotho, Yzeworth, Xoro, Quotwe, Theosy, Meweth, Xosoy, Yachyros, Gaba, Hagay, Staworo, Wyhaty, Ruoso Xuatho, Rum, Ruwoth, Zyros, Quaylos, Wewor, Vegath, Wysor, Wuzoy, Noses, * Aziel.*

✠　　　✠　　　✠

ARIELIS

Seal or Character for Coercion and Obedience.

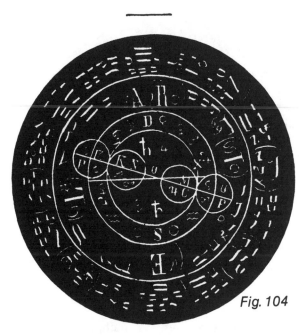

Fig. 104

Yschiros, Theor Zebaoth, Wyzeth, Yzathos, Xyzo, Xywethoror-woy, Xantho, Wiros, Rurawey, Ymowe, Noswathosway, Wuvnetho-wesy, Zebaoth, Yvmo, Zvswethonowe, Yschyrioskay, Ulathos, Wyzoy, Yrsawo, Xyzeth, Durobijthaos, Wuzowethus, Yzweoy, Zaday, Zywaye, Hagathorwos, Yachyros, Imas, Tetragrammaton, Ariel.

Citation of Marbuel

✠   ✠   ✠

MARBUELIS

Seal or Character for Coercion and Obedience.

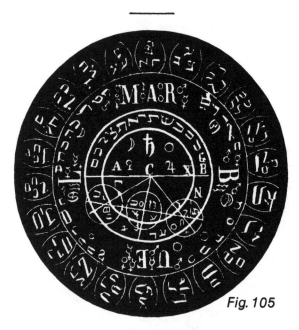

Fig. 105

Adonay, Jehova, Zebaoth, Theos, Yzhathoroswe, Wehozymathos, Zosim, Yghoroy, Vegorym, Abaij, Wogos, Gijghijm, Zeowoij, Ykosowe, Wothym, Kijzwe, Uijwoth, Omegros, Hehgewe, Zebaoij, Wezator, Zibuo, Sijbetho, Ythos, Zeatijm, Wovoe, Sijwoijmwethij, Pharvoij, Zewor, Wegfos, Ruhen, Hvbathoroos, Stawows, Zijen, Zijwowij, Haros, Worse, Yzwet, Zebaoth, Agla, Marbuel.

✠ ✠ ✠

MEPHISTOPHILIS

Seal of Character for Coercion and Obedience

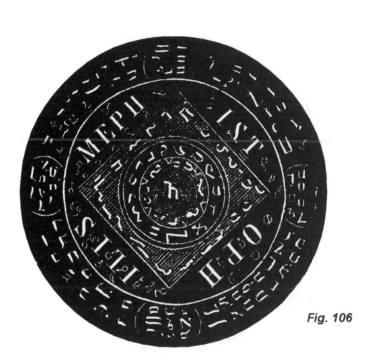

Fig. 106

Messias, Adonaij, Weforus, Xathor, Yxewe, Soraweijs, Yxaron, Wegharh, Zijhalor, Weghaij, Weosron, Xoxijwe, Zijwohwawetho, Ragthoswatho, Zebaoth, Adonaij, Zijwetho, Aglaij, Wiizathe, Zadaij, Zijebo, Xosthoy, Athlato, Zsewey, Zyxyset, Ysche, Sarsewu, Zyzym, Deworonhathbo, Xyxewe, Syzwe, Theos, Yschaos, Worsonbefgosy, Gefgowe, Hegor, Quaratho, Zywe, Messias, Abarabi, Mephistophilis.

✠ ✠ ✠

BARBUELIS

Seal of Character for Coercion and Obedience

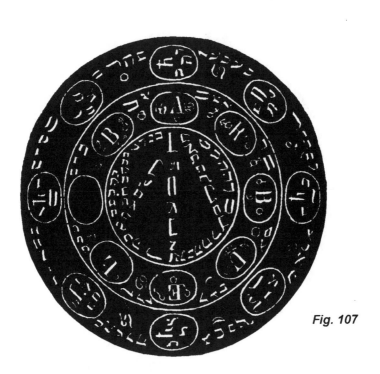

Fig. 107

Yschiros, Imns, Zebaoth, Otheos, Kuwethosorym, ZylohynZaday, Yschowe, Quyos, Zenhatorowav, Yzwesor, Xywoy, Yzyryr,Zalijmo, Zabaoth, Adonaii, Messias, Aglabaij, Stoweos, Hijwetho,Ycoros, Zijwetho, Uwoim, Chamoweo, Zijzobeth, Sotho, Emnohalj, Zedije, Huwethos, Chorij, Yzquoos, Liraije, Weghoijm, Xiixor, Waijos, Gofaljme, Toroswe, Yeijros, Emanuel, Imas, Barbuel.

Citation of Aziabel

✠   ✠   ✠

AZIABELIS

Seal of Character for Coercion and Obedience

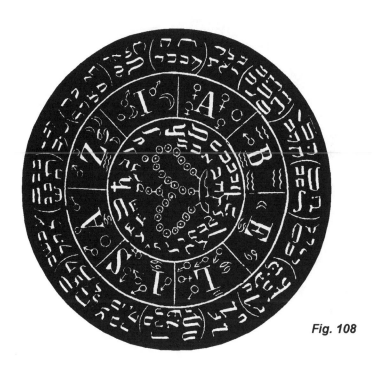

Fig. 108

Thoeos, Ygweto, Yzgowoij, Quiseo, Wijzope, Xorsoij, Nowetho, Yxose, Haguthou, Xoro, Theos, Magowo, Wijzosorwothe, Xaroshaij, Zebaoth, Emanuel, Messias, Yzijwotho, Zadaij, Xexhatosiimeij, Buwatho, Ysewet, Xijrathor, Zijbos, Malhaton, Yzos, Uzewor, Raguil, Wewot, Yzewewe, Quorhijm, Zadob, Zibathor, Weget, Zijzawe, Ulijzor, Tetragrammaton, Aziabel.

Citation of Anituel

✠   ✠   ✠

ANTQUELIS

Seal of Character for Coercion and Obedience

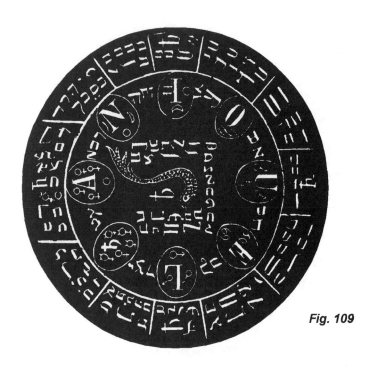

Fig. 109

Thoeos, Aba, Aaba, Aba, Agathoswaij, Yzoroij, Ywetho, Quardos, Quasoai, Uschjjros, Cijmce, Qowathim, Geofoli, Zarobe, Weghatj, Ohegathorowaij, Mesows, Xalose, Waghthorsowe, Wephatho, Yzebo, Storilwethonaij, Quorathon, Sijbo, Mephor, Wijhose, Zaloros, Ruetho, Zebaathonaijwos, Zijweth, Ycarij, Ruwethonowe, Ruiathosowaij, Zebaoth, Messias, Anituel.

THE USE OF THE SEALS

If these great princes do not appear immediately on the foregoing Citations, or if they hesitate in their obedience, then cast frankincense and myrh upon burning coals; when the smoke arises, place the spirit seal thereon, and pronounce the following mysterious words:

ALTISSIMA DIE VERBA

Spirituum Cactiva Mosis Aaron et Salomonis

Zijmuorsobet, Noijm, Zavaxo, Quehaij, Abawo, Noquetonaij, Oasaij, Wuram, Thefotoson, Zijoronoaifwetho, Mugelthor, Yzxe, Agiopuaij, Huzije, Surhatijm, Sowe, Oxursoij, Zijbo, Yzweth, Quaij, Salrthos, Quaij, Qeahaij, Qijrpu, Sardowe, Xoro, Wuggofhoswerhiz, Kaweko, Ykquos, Zehatho, Aba. Amen.

The Apparition

The conjured spirit will appear almost as soon as these word are said. As soon as he appears, address and compel him with the following words.

Binding Of Moses

Zebaoth, Abatho, Tetragrammaton, Adonaij, Abathoij, Zijhawe, Aglaij, Quohowe, Agla, Muijroshoweth, Phalowaij, Agla, Theos, Messias, Zijwethororijm, Feghowo, Aba, Mowewo, Choe, Adonaij, Cewoe, Christohatos, Tetragrammaton.

Instructions

Since the spirits will now appear quickly, express your desires to them clearly, honestly and without fear for nothing can harm you. Rather they must serve you obediently and give your all you require of them. However, remember not to compromise with any spirits in any way, do not yield to them in any way, and be firm in your demeanor. For these words of might and power that you have used in the conjuration are sufficient to compel the spirits to obey you and to do so without harm or deception.

MIHI FAUSTO † EXPERTO

VALEDICTO OR DISMISSAL OF THE SPIRITS

Since the spirits have now served you according to your wishes, dismiss them and discharge them with the following words:

Zebaoth, Theos, Yschyres, Messias, Imas, Weghaymnko, Quoheos, Roveym, Christoze, Abay, Xewefaraym, Agla.

And now depart in the name of God. Praise, love and thank God to the end.

8. The Rabellini Table or Tabellae Rabellinae

for the

Command of Spirits

General Citation of White and Black Magic for the Invocation of Good and Evil Spirits

Roma, Vaticano ad Arcanum Pontificatus Under Pope Alexander VI

Printed in 1501 A.D.

EDITOR'S NOTE:

The Citation, Coercion and Dismission of Spirits given in the Rabellini Table can be used to invoke, bind and dismiss all spirits, be they good or evil. A small list of the spirits who can be conjured through this table follows.

Monarchy of the Good and Familiar Spirits

The following angelic spirits can be cited for all human ministrations: Seraphim Uriel, Cherubim Raphael, Thronus Oriphiel, Dominatio Zachariel, Potestas Gabriel, Virtus Barbiel, Principatus Requel, Archangelus Anael, Angelus Phaleg.

These are the Princes of the nine Choir of Angels. They have among them many spirits 1,000 times 1,000 without end. Sanctus, Sanctus, Sanctus.

These angelic spirits appear very willingly to human beings to help and serve them in all things.

Other Good Spirits

Chymchy, Asbeor, Yzazel, Xomoy, Asmoy, Diema, Bethor, Arfose, Zenay, Corowe, Orowor, Xonor, Quilheth, Quato, Wewor, Gefowe, Gorhon, Woreth, Hagyr, Welor.

Archarontica or Evil Spirits

Even though evil, the following spirits are still familiar or ministering spirits, and are ready to serve.

Thebot, Wethor, Quorthonn, Ywote, Yrson, Xysorym, Zuwoy, Puchon, Tulef, Legioh, Xexor, Woryon.

Instructions

Concerning white magic, take notice that all good spirits must be cited when the moon is full, the Princes of the nine Choir of Angels, as well as the other good spirits.

Concerning black magic, take notice that the Seven Princes of Evil must be cited during new moon. Other evil spirits are cited most readily in the dark of the moon, or at the time of an eclipse of the sun or the moon. The circle already given in Fig. 102, as coercive of hell, is to be used for all spirits, good or evil.

General Citation of Moses, Aaron and Solomon for All Spirits

Aba, Alpha, Omega, Hewozywetony, Xewerator, Menhatoy, Queo, Zuwezet, Rumoy, Ruwetze, Quano, Duzy, Zenthono-Rohmatru, Xono, Zonozebethoos, Zebaoth, Aglay, Tetragrammaton, Adonay, Theos, Ysehyroroseth, Zumquvos, Nywe, Athanatos, Thoy, Quyhet, Homor, Wethoum, Ywae, Ysgeboth, Oray, Zywo, Ysgewot, Zururogos, Zuy, Zywethorosto, Rurom, Xuwye, Xunewe, Keoso, Wecato, Zyweso, Tetragrammaton.

Now pronounce the name of the good or evil +++ spirit distinctly that you wish to conjure. He will appear very suddenly. You then may address him.

Coercion or Binding Of Spirits

Theohatatos, Quyseym, Gefgowe, Phagayr, Messias. Amen.

Valedictio or Dismissal of Spirits

Theos, Zebaoth, Adonay, Ischiros, Zaday, Messias, Salomos, Yweth, Thors, Yzheto, Thyym, Quowe, Xehatoym, Phoe, Tetragrammaton.

Now pronounce the name of the spirit and let him depart in peace. Deus Principium et Finis.

PART III

THE SEMIPHORAS
AND
SCHEMHAMPHORAS

EDITOR'S NOTE:

The Semiphoras are names of God, some of them lengthy, through which many wondrous things can be accomplished, according to the Hebrew magical tradition. There are usually seven Semiphoras, each one used for a different purpose. In this work two versions of the Semiphoras are given. In the first version, the seven Semiphoras of Adam are described, and the holy names given in detail. In the second version, the seven Semiphoras of Moss are discussed, and the holy names given, together with their traditional uses.

The Schemhamphoras, on the other hand, is a name of God containing seventy-two letters. It is the most powerful of the names of the Deity, according to tradition, and its secrets are hidden in Chapter XIV of Exodus in the original Hebrew version. Those readers interested to learn more about the Schempham-phoras or Kabbalah in general are directed to this editor's work, A Kabbalah for the Modern World, which deals with the subject in detail.

SEMIPHORAS AND SCHEHAMPHORAS

King Solomon

Wesel, Duisburg and Frankfurt

Printed and Published by Andrew Luppius, Licensed Publisher

in the above cities

1686

1. Prayer and Explanation

An Humble Prayer for the Attainment of Wisdom and Understanding

"For the lord giveth wisdom, out of his mouth cometh knowledge and understanding." (Proverbs 2:6).

If any of you lack wisdom let him ask of God, that giveth to all men liberally, and upbraideth not." (Epistle of James 1:5)

Oh, God my Father and Lord of all goodness, who didst create all things by Thy word, and who didst prepare man in thy wisdom to rule over all creatures that were made by Thee, that he should rule over the world with holiness and righteousness, and judge with an upright heart. Give unto me that wisdom that is constantly around Thy throne, and cast me not out from among Thy children. For I am Thy servant, and the child of Thine handmaiden, a weak creature of a short existence, and too weak in understanding, in right and in the law. Send it down from Thy high heaven and from the throne of Thy glory that it may abide with me and labor with me, that I may know and do the things that are pleasing unto Thee. For Thy wisdom knoweth and understandeth all things, and let it lead me in my works and protect me in its glory, and my labors will be acceptable unto Thee. When I was yet in my youth I sought wisdom without fear in my prayer. I prayed for it in the temple, and will seek it to my end. My heart rejoiceth over it as when the young grapes ripen. Thou art my Father, my God and my Shepherd, who helpest me. Thy hand created and prepared me. Teach me that I may learn Thy commandements. Open my eyes that I may behold the wonders of Thy law. Remember, Lord, Thy covenant, and teach me what to say and think. Instruct me and so shall I live. Lord, show me Thy ways, lead me in Thy truth, and teach me. I am Thy servant, teach me that I may understand Thy evidence. Console me again with Thy help and let the happy spirit sustain me. Thou lover of life, Thy immortal spirit is in all things. Teach me to work in a manner that is well pleasing unto Thee, for Thou art my God. Let Thy good spirit lead me in pleasant paths. With Thee is the living fontain and in Thy light we see the light. Let my goings be established, and let no unrighteousness rule over me. Teach me wholesome manners and enlighten me, for I believe Thy commandments. Lead me in Thy truth and teach me, for Thou art the God who helps me, and I wait daily before Thee. Let Thy countenance shine upon Thy servant and teach me to know Thy justice. Let me behold Thy glory, for Thou, Lord, art my light, and Thou wilt turn my darkness into day. Wilt Thou join Thyself with me in eternity, and trust me in righteousness and judgment, in grace and mercy, yea, wilt Thou join me in faith that I may know Thee, the Lord. Lord, let my complaints come before Thee. Instruct me according to Thy word. Let my prayers come before Thee, rescue me according to Thy word. Show me Thy ways, Oh Lord, that I may walk in Thy truth. Keep my heart in singleness that I may fear Thy name. I will remember Thy name from childhood. Therefore all people will thank Thee forever and ever. Amen-

Explanation by King Solomon

In the name of the highest Almighty Creator, I, King Solomon, hold to the interpretation of the name of (God) Semiphoras, in other words, the First and the Greatest, the oldest and hidden mystery of great power and virtue. To obtain all that which is asked of God, He must be worshipped in spirit and in truth because each word and name of God is self-existent. Therefore the name and the prayer must agree and no strange name must be used unnecessarily. The consciousness of God in His name (through which He comes near) abides with those who know His name. Therefore this nam must be held in the highest honor and hidden from all frivolous and unworthy persons, since God says Himself in Exodus: Out of all places will I come unto thee and bless thee because thou rememberest my name. Therefore have the Hebrew Maccabees seventy-two names for God, and named and wrote Schemhaphoras, the name of seventy-Two letters.

First, it must be known that the names of God cannot be taught and understood except in the Hebrew language. Neither can we pronounce them in any other dialect, as they were revealed to us through the grace of God. Forthey are the sacrament and emanation of divine omnipotence, not of man, nor of angels, but they are instituted and consecrated through God, to instill divine harmony in a certain manner according to the characters of his immovable number and figure, and of which those that are appointed over the heavens are afraid. The angels and all creatures honor them and use them to praise their Creator and to bless Him with the greatest reverence in His divine works. Whosoever will apply them properly with fear and trembling and with prayer, will be powerfully enlightened by the Spirit of God, will be joined with a divine unity, will be mighty according to the will of God that he can perform supernatural things, that he can command angels and devils, that he can bind and unbind the things of the elements, over which he may elevate himself through the power of God. Therefore, he, who has purified and improved his understanding and morals, and who, through faith, has purified his ears, so that he may without spurious alterations call upon the divine name of God, will become a house and a dwelling place of God, and will be a partaker of divine influences.

Second, the order of God should be known, that God makes use of certain words among angels and certain others maong men. However, the true name of God is known neither to men nor to angels, for He has reserved it, and will not reveal it until His order and exhibition are perfected. Then the angels will have their own tongue and speech, about which we need not concern ourselves because it is not necessary for us to examine them.

Third, all the names of God are taken by us from His works, as an indication of a communication with Him, or are extracted from the scriptures through the art of the Kabbalah.

The beginning of the name and word Semiphoras, which God the Creator, Jehovah, gave in Paradise, embraces three Hebrew letters, Jehovah the Inscrutable Creator of the World, Almighty Providence, and All-Powerful Strong Diety.

There are four parts of the earth which are the most subtle light of the spiritual world. They are, Cherubim et Seraphim; Potestates et Virtutes; Archangelos et Angelos; and Spiritus et Hominum, which come before God. This part of the world also has four angels that stand upon the four corners of heaven. They are Michael, Raphael, Gabriel and Uriel. Four angels also stand for the elements, namely, Seraph, Cherub, Tharsis and Ariel.

The heavens is divided into four triplicities, that is, three zodiacal signs for each of the four elements, fire, water, air, and earth. These triplicities form twelve zodiac signs under which the sun revolves yearly, marking the change of seasons and changing the fourth element.

Man has four elements within him. Anima is in the head; Spiritus is in the heart and operates through the arteries; Corpus is the whole body, acting with the veins; Genius, a spark of fire, is in the kidneys and rules birth. Man also has four spiritual working faculties known as Animali, Vitalis, Naturalis, and Genitions. The soul has inward senses in which faith acts and other intellectual senses in the brain.

Imaginatrix, the imagination, is another soul operation which draws a picture of power and accomplishes all things. Rativtanatio repeats the species on the mind on all cause and judgments. If the soul turns to real reason, it will obtain a knowledge of all worldly wisdom. Lastly, memoratrix, or memory, retains all things which pertain to the faculties and operations of the spirit. Through agitation of the nerves the increase of the human race is effected by God. The living spirit of the heart embraces within itself four virtues: Justice, Temperance, Prudence and Fortitude. These lie in the arterial blood and connect the soul with the body. The natural spiritual action and power lies in the liver and arteries and effect motion and attraction, support and subsistence. The proper spirit of strength and sap lies in the kidneys to multiply through divine perfection.

In the four quarter of the world there is darkness, instituted for condemnation in wrath and for punishment. Four princes of devils are injurious in the four elements: Samael, Azazel, Azael, Mehazaer. Four princes of devils rule over the four quarters of the earth: Oriens, Pagmon, Egyn, Amayon.

The Seven Semiphoras of Adam

The first Semiphoras is that of Adam because he spoke with God, the Creator, in Paradise.

The second Semiphoras because he spoke with angels and spirits

The third because he spoke with devils.

The fourth because he spoke with the creatures of the four elements, the birds, the fish, the animals, and the creeping things of the earth.

The fifth because he spoke with inanimate objects, such as herbs, seeds, trees and all vegetation.

The sixth because he spoke with the winds.

The seventh because he spoke with the sun, the moon and the stars.

By the power of the seven semiphoras he could create and destroy all he desired.

The first Semiphoras was acknowledged by Adam since God created him and placed him in Paradise, where he was allowed to remain only seven hours. The name of the first Semiphoras is Jove and it must only be pronounced in the greatest need, and then only with the most devout feelings toward the Creator. In this case you will find grace and sure help.

The second Semiphoras in which Adam spoke with the angels, an which is Yeseraye, that is, God without Beginning and Without End, must be pronounced when speaking with angels. Then your questions will be answered and your wishes fulfilled.

The third Semiphoras, through which Adam spoke with the spirits of the departed, is Adonay Saboath, cadas Adonay amara. These words must be uttered when one wishes to collect winds, spirits or demons, Aly, Adoy, Sabaoth, amara.

The fourth Semiphoras is Layamen, Iava, firi, Iavagellayn, Lavaquiri, Lavagola, Lavatasorin, Layfialafin, Lyafaran. With this name he bound and unbound all animals and spirits.

The fifth Semiphoras is Lyacham, Lyalgema, Lyafarau, Lialfarah, Lebara, Lebarosin, Layararalus. If you wish to bind treese and seeds, must pronounce the above words.

The sixth Semiphoras is great in might and virtue. It is Letamnin, Letaylogo, Letasynin, Levaganaritin, Letarminin, Letagelogin, Lotafalosin. Use these when you desire the elements or winds to fulfil your wishes.

The seventh Semiphoras is great and mighty. These are the names of the Creator, which must be pronounced at the beginning of each undertaking. Eliaon yoena Adonay cadas ebreel, eloy ela agiel, ayoni, Sachado, essuselas eloyrn, delion iau elynla, delia, yazi, Zazael, paliel man, umiel, onela dilatan saday alma paneim alym, canal deus Usami yaras calipix calfas sasna saffasaday aylata panteomel auriel arion phaneton secare panerionys emanel Joth Jalaph amphia, than demisrael mu all le Leazyns ala phonar aglacyei qyol paeriteron theferoym barimel, jael haryon ya apiolell ehcet.

These holy names must be pronounced each time in reverence toward God when you desire to accomplish something through the elements or connected with them. Your wishes will then be fulfilled, what is to be destroyed will be destroyed, for God will be with you because you know His name.

The Seven Semiphoras of Moses

The following is another name of Semiphoras that God gave to Moses in seven parts.

The first Semiphoras was given to Moses when he spoke with God in the Burning Bush.

The second, when he spoke with God, the Creator, on the mountain.

The Third, when he divided the Red Sea, and passed through with the people of Israel.

The fourth, when his staff was turned into a serpent in Pharoah's court.

The fifth are the names which were written on Aaron's forehead.

The sixth was given to Moses when he made a brazen serpent and burned the golden calf to divert pestilence from the Israelites.

The seventh, when manna fell down from heaven in the wilderness and water gushed from the rock.

In the first Semiphoras are found the words which Moses spake as he spoke to the fire in the Burning Bush. They are: Maya, Affaby, Zien, Jaramye, yne Latebni damaa yrsano, noy lyloo lhay yly yre Eylvi Zya Lyelee, Loate, lideloy eyloy, mecha ramethy rybifassa fu aziry schihiu rite Zelohabe vete hebe ede neyo ramy rahabe (conoc anuhec). If you pray this word to God devoutly, your undertaking will be fulfilled without a doubt.

In the second Semiphoras are the words which God spake to Moses as he went up the mountain. They are: Abtan, Abynistan, Zoratan Juran nondieras, potarte faijs alapeina pognij podaij sacroficium. In these words the prophet spoke to the angels with whom the four quarters of the earth are sealed, through which the the temple was founded Bosale. If you wish to pronounce these words, you should fast three days, be chaste and pure, and then you can perform many wonders.

In the third Semiphoras are words which Moses spake in order to divide the Red Sea: Oua claiie saijec holomomaatl; bekahn aijclo inare asnia haene hieha ijfale malieha arnija aremeholona queleij, Lineno feijano, ijoije malac habona nethee hijcere. If you have lost favor of your master, or if you wish to gain the good will of someone, speak these words with fervor and humility.

In the fourth Semiphoras are the words which Moses spoke when he changed his staff into a serpent: Micrato, raepijsathonich petanith pistan ijtn ijer hijgarin ijgnition temayron aijcon dunsnas casta Laciaastas ijecon cijna caihera natu facas. Pronounce these names when you wish to have your desires fulfilled.

In the fifth Semiphoras are the names written on Aaron's forehead as he spake with the Creator: Sadaij haijlves Lucas elacijus jaconi hasihaia ijein ino, sep, actitas barne lud doncnij eijaiehhu reu, vaha, vialia, eije. Vie haija hoij asaija salna hahai, ˙ cuci ijaija. Elenehel, na vena; setna. The names are powerful in satisfying each request.

In the sixth Semiphoras are the names written upon Moses' staff, when he made the brazen serpent and broke the golden calf. They are: Tane mare syam, abijl ala, nuno, hija actenal tijogas ijano, eloim ija nehn ijane haij ijanehn, ahijaco, mea. With this name destroy all sorcery and evil. You must not pronounce it with levity in your works.

In the seventh Semiphoras are the words which Moses employed in leading the Israelites out of Egypt, with which he brought manna from heaven and caused water to flow from the rock: Sadaij amara elon pheneton eloij eneij ebeoel messias ijahe vehu hejiane, ijanancl elijon. Pronounce these words when you desire to do something wonderful, or when you are in great need, and call earnestly on God.

Prayer

Oh, thou living God. Thou great, strong, mighty , holy and pure Creator full of mercy - a blessed Lord of all things. Praised be Thy name. I implore Thee, fulfill my desire. Thou canst work. Permit us to accomplish this work. Grant us Thy grace and give us Thy divine blessing, that we may happily fulfill this work. Thou holy, merciful and gracious God, have mercy upon us. Thy name, Jeseraire be adored forever and ever. Amen.

In the name of the Almighty Creator, I, Solomon, hold to the declaration of the divine name, Agla. Thou are a mighty God to all eternity. He who bears upon his person this name, written upon a gold plate, will never die a sudden death. Ararita - a beginning of all unity. Ahen - Thou solid rock, united with the Son. Amen. Thou. Lord, a true King, perfect.

The names consist of the beginning of the chapter Adonay, which the Hebrews used instead of the unutterable name Asser Eserie.

The seven mighty names may be obtained at a favorable hour and place. They are: Comiteijon, sede aij, throtomas, sasmagata bij ijl ijcos.

The four names of the Creator are: Jva, Jona, eloij, Jeua. He who calls often upon God in faith and with fear, and carries with him the golden letters, will never want for an honorable subsistence and good clothing.

The name which Adam uttered at the entrance to hell is: mephenaij phaton. He who carries this name with him is unconquerable.

The name which God communicated to Moses on Mount Sinai, Hacedion, will put away all causes of sorrow.

The name wich Joshua prayed when the sun stood still, baahando heltaloir, dealzhat, brings vengeance upon enemies.

The ten names of the Sephiroth, which I, Solomon, spoke in may prayer to God, and though which he gave me wisdom are: Kether, Hochmah, Binah, Chesed, Geburah, Tiphereth, Netzach, Hod, Yesod, and Malkuth.

The ten names of God are: Eheie, Yod Tetragrammaton, Tetragrammaton Sabaoth, Elohim Sabaoth, Sadaij Adonaij nulech, all with then letters in the original Hebrew. Tretragrammaton Vedath have eight letters. Eheie, the self-existence of God, Arerite Aser Eheie, are the names of God of seven letters.

Eseh, used by Moses as the Fire of God, Elion, has five letters and they are all Hebrew characters.

Emeth, the true God, is God's seal. The explanation of the ten names of God and the ten Sephiroth, is given by Cornelius Agrippa in his work, De Occulta Philsophia.

Hacaba, the holy and adored God.

Hu, himself the power of the Deity.

Hod, Yod, a divine being.

Jah, a just God, comparing himself with man.

Inon.

Jesuba, the Messiah will come in the golden age.

Jaua, he who created the light.

Isaia, with the name El, resembles the changed era (each made up of 31).

Mettratron for Sadai, each name composed of 314 characters.

Icuru Maapaz, both names are derived from a transposition of the name Jehovah.

Messiah is derived from a transposition of the letters in Jisma Macom.

Na, the name of God, should be used in tribulation and oppression.

Oromasim, Mitrim, Araminem signify God and the Spirit. They are three princes of the world.

Pele, he who worketh wonders.

These names must be selected out of each letter constituting the work, for the accomplishment of which the help of God should be implored.

The name of God of seventy-two letters is hidden in a certain part of Exodus, Chapter 14. The name consists of three verses which are always written with seventy-two letters, beginning with the three words: Vaijsa, Vaiduo, Vaiot, which, when placed on a line, one and three, from left to right, the middle one transposed from the right to the left, a name of God is formed, the seventy-two letters of which are called the Schemhamphoras.

The
Schemhamforas

Which will certainly bring to light the Treasures of Earth,
if buried in the Treasure - Earth

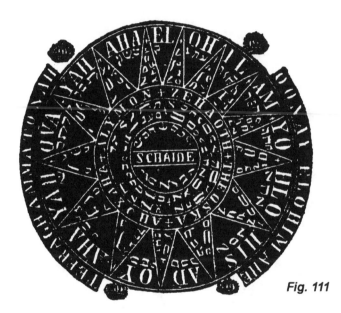

Fig. 111

From the Arcan Bible of Moses

From
P. Hoffman, Jesuit
Composed ad Proxim
L. MISCHINSKY, at RAOL, MDCCXLVL

SCHEMHAMFORAS
No. 1

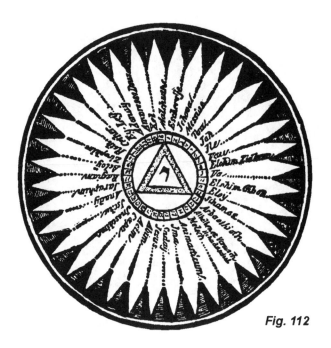

Fig. 112

Seu septuaginta duo Divina Nomina in lingua Hebraic, denotant semper
Nomen deisive legantur a principo fine veladextrisant sonistris suntque
ingentis virtutis.

SCHEMHAMFORAS

No. 2

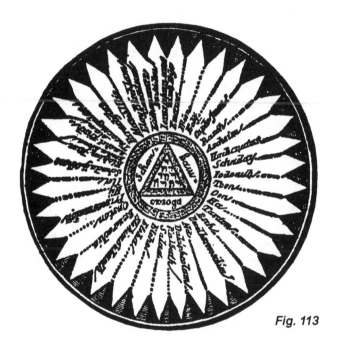

Fig. 113

If the divine names, El or Jad, are then added, there will be seventy-two names of God, each of them syllables, for it is written: My angel goeth before me, behold him, for my name is in him. There are seventy-two deacons of the five departments of heaven; there are so many nations and tongues, so many bodily functions working with the seventy-two disciples of Christ. And this is one method used by the Kabbalists in making up these names.

Another method used to form the Schemhamphoras is by writing the three verses in regular order from right to left, without selecting this method from the Tables of Zimph, or as it is selected from the Table of Commutations.

Vehuiah, Jeliel, Sitael, Elemiah, Mahasia, Lehalel, Achuiah, Cahetel, Haziel, Aladiah, Laviah, Caliel, Leuniah, Pahaliah, Nelchael, Leiaiel, Melahel, Hahuiah, Mittaiah, Haaiah, Jerathel, Scehia, Rauel, Omael, Lecabel, Vasarias, Jehujah, Labahiah, Chauakiah, Mahadel, Aniel, Haamiah, Richael, Ieiazcl, Hahael, Michael, Vehuel, Daniel, Hahasias, Imamiahs, Nanael, Nitael, Behahia, Poiel, Nemamiah; Selalel, Harael, Mizrael, Sahhel, Annanuel, Mehael, Damabiah, Menkiel, Eliapel, Habuiah, Rochel, Jabamiah, Haianel, Maniah.

In the first period of nature, God was addressed by the name of Sadai Trigrammaton. In the second period of the Law, he bore the unutterable name of Tetragrammaton, which is substituted by the name Adonaij. In the period of grace he was called Pentagrammaton effabile Jesu, which is also written Jusu, with four letters, and JHS with three letters.

The Father gave all power to the Son, the angels received heaven, but the name of God and Jesus, who is the first power in God. Afterwards it spread to the twelve and the seven angels, through which it was communicated to the twelve zodiacal signs and the seven planets, and consequently, to all the servants and instruments of God. Jesus said: Everything which ye ask of the Father in my name, that he will give unto you, if ye pray unto him with a pure heart and a fervent spirit, for there is no other name given to man whereby he can be saved but the name of Jesus. Amen.

2. Of the Benefit and Uses of the Semiphoras

With humility, faith and trust in the Creator, man must implore divine help and blessing, praying fervently and continuously, that God may enlighten the mind, and take away from the soul all the darkness of the material body. For when our soul is moved by a special cause, it also moves the various parts of the body to work towards the accomplishment of our desires. Therefore, the great Creator, when He is worshipped in spirit and in truth, and when no unecessary things are asked of Him, when the prayer is devoutly expressed, will cause the lower order of creatures to yield obedience to the wishes of man, according to their state, order and calling. Man was made in the image and likeness of God and endowed with reason through the favor of God, and he will obtain his desires through faith and wisdom. First, from the stars and from the heavens by the rational reflections of His spirit; second, by the animal kingdom, through man's own senses; and third, by the elements, through man's fourfold body.

Therefore, man binds all creatures by calling upon the higher power, through the name and power which governs one thing, and thereafter through the lower things themselves.

And now, he who desires to become master of the workings of the soul, must become familiar with the order of all things, just as they are obtained by God in their proper state, from the highest to the lowest, through natural connections, that he may descend as if from a ladder. On this account, the heathen nations committed the error of worshipping the planets and the stars, not realizing that these forces were moved and influenced by the Creator of all. The

Christian nations also erred in paying homage to departed saints and giving honor to creatures who belong to the Creator. And God is a jealous God and will not permit the worship of idols. The prayer of faith, therefore, in proper language and for proper objects, is intimately related to the name of God, from which we descent by words, from one to the other, following each other out of a natural relationship, in order to accomplish something.

He who desires the influence of the sun, must not only direct his eyes towards it, but he must also elevate his soul power to the soul power of the sun, which is God Himself. Such a person must have previously made himself equal to God through fasting, purification and good works. He must also pray in the name of the Mediator, with fervent love to God and his fellow man, that he may come to the sun spirit, so that he may be filled with its light and luster, which he may draw himself from heaven, and that he may become gifted with heavenly powers and obtain all the desires of his heart. As soon as he grasps the higher light and arrives at a state of perfection, being gifted with supernatural intelligence, he will also obtain supernatural might and power. For this reason, without Godliness, man will deny Christ and will become unacceptable to God, therewith falling prey to the evil spirits against whom there is no better protection than the fear of the Lord and fervent love of God and man.

Most people who are skilled in divine works, and who possess the right to command spirits, must be worthy by nature or become worthy by education and discipline for their calling. They must also keep all their works secret, but must not conceal them from truly pious persons.

If a man has knowledge of God as the first great cause, he must also acknowledge other causes or cooperative spirits, and determine what dignity and honor to accord them. Without this knowledge their presence and help cannot be enjoyed. Such honor and dignity must not be shown for the sake of the spirits themselves, but for the sake of their Lord, whose servants they are. In this manner the angels of God will gather around those who fear and love the Lord.

The Hebrew Kabbalists and theologians named ten divine names as members of God, and ten Numerations or Sephiroth as raiments and instruments of the Creator, through which He is infused into all His creatures according to the order of the Ten Angelic and ten Princely Spirit Choirs, from which all things derive their existence. The divine names and their numbers or Sephiroth follow.

1. The name EHEIE ASER EHEIE, whose number and Sephiroth is Kether Elion, one Lord, is the simplest Deity, whom no eye has seen at any time. It is ascribed to God the Father, gives influence through the order Seraphim Haiath Heiadosch, gate of holiness or of life, that transmits life to everything through Elieic. From this He flows in through the Premium Mobile so that all things will come into being. This wonderful being is called Intelligentsia Mettraton, that is, a Prince of Faces. His office is to lead others into the presence of the Divine Sovereign. Through him God spake to Moses.

2. The name JEHOVAH, JOD VEL JAH, whose number or Sephiroth is Hochmah, that is, Wisdom, or the Deity full of Spirit. The firstborn son through whom the Father redeemed man from his curse, is infused through the order of Cherubim, in Hebrew Orphanim, of te form or Council. From these He flows into the heavens where he produces many forms. This is God, Jod, Tetragrammaton, through the peculiar Intelligentsia Razielem, who was a representative of Adam.

3. The name TETRAGRAMMATON ELOHIM, whose number and Sephiroth is called Binah, that is, Understanding, caution or sense. It signifies pardon and rest, cheerfulness, repentance and conversion. It is the great trumpet, the redemption of the world and life in time to come. It is adapted to the Holy Spirit and flows in its might through the order of Thronum, which is called Arabim in Hebrew, that is, the great, strong and mighty angels, who flow through the Saturn sphere and give liquid matter the form Stopsie, which was

the Intelligentsia Zaphekiel, Noah's representative. It is also the Intelligentsia Jophiel, Shem's representative. These are the three highest and greatest Numerations, the throne of Divinity, through whose commands everything takes place. The following seven Numerations or Sepiroth are called Numerationes Fabrice.

4. The name El, whose number or Sephiroth is Chesed, that is, grace or goodness. It is called Mercy, pity, great power, sceptre, and right hand, and flows through the order of the Dominations, in Hebrew Chasmalin. It confers peaceable justice through the Jupiter Sphere and bestows the special Intelligentsia Zadkiel, Abraham's representative.

5. The name ELOHIM GEBOR, whose number or Sephiroth is Geburah, that is, might, gravity, strength, severity, security, judgment. This is a strong God, who punishes the guilty and the wicked. He inflicts punishment through the sword and through wars. To this is added the Judgment seat of God, the girdle of the Lord, a sword and left arm. It is also Pached, that is, fear before God. It flows through the order of the Potestats, in Hebrew Seraphim. From thence through the Mars sphere, which brings great wars and tribulation and moves the elements accordingly. Its peculiar Intelligentsia is Gamael, Samson's representative.

6. The name is ELOHA, the God of Alchemy, and its number or Sephiroth is Tiphereth, that is, beauty, adornment, happiness and pleasure. It signifies the world of life and flows through the Order of Virtues, in Hebrew Malachim. This angel, through the Sun sphere, gives perspicuity and life, and reveals metals. His peculiar Intelligentsia, Raphael, was Isaac's representative and also Tobias'. Pehel was Jacob's representative.

7. The name is TRETRAGRAMMATON SABAOTH, whose number or Sephiroth is Netzach, that is, triumph and victory. It is also called Adonay Sabaoth, God of Hosts. This name signifies eternity, the justice of God and His avenger. He flows through the Order of Principatum, in Hebrew Elohim, that is, God in the Venus sphere,

which is love and joy. He produces all vegetable growth and His peculiar intelligentsia is Hanael. The angel Cernaiul is David's representative.

8. The name is ELOHIM SABAOTH, God of Hosts, not of war or wrath, but of pity, for He has both names and goes before his hosts. His number and Sephiroth is Hod, that is, honorable confession, ornament and renown. He flows through the order of Archangels and the Mercury sphere. He brings forth animals. His peculiar intelligentsia is Michael, Solomon's representative.

9. The name is SADAI, the Almighty, who doeth all things abundantly. His number and Sephiroth is Yesod, that is, foundation, and is denominated good sense, redemption and rest. He flows through the order of Angels, in Hebrew Cherubim, and the Moon sphere, to increase and decrease all things. It supports and contributes the genius of man. His intelligentsia is Gabriel, a representative of Joseph, Joshua and Daniel.

10. The name is ADONAY MELECH, that is, a Lord and a King. His number and Sephiroth is Malkuth, that is, a kingdom and a dominion. It is termed the church and house of God and the door through which it flows is the order of Animasticum of the believing soul; in Hebrew, the life of princes. They give information to the children of men about all wonderful things and guard them against prophecies. Their anima Messiah Meschia (and the intelligentsia Mettraton, which is called the first creature and soul of the world) is Moses' representative.

The nine choirs of angels, or according to Dionysius, the ten blessed orders, are:

1. Seraphim

2. Cherubim

3. Thrones

4. Dominationis

5. Potestates

6. Virtues

7. Principalities

8. Archangels

9. Angels

10. Blessed Souls

The Hebrews called them by the following names:

1. Chaioth

2. Hacades

3. Ophanim

4. Aralim

5. Chasmalin

6. Seraphim

7. Malachim Elohim

8. Ben Elohim

9. Cherubim

10. Issim

The ten representative angels are:

1. Mettraton
2. Jophiel
3. Zaphkiel
4. Camael
5. Raphael
6. Haniel
7. Michael
8. Gabriel
9. Ratziel
10. Anima Messiah

3. On the Hierarchy of Angels

In the first hierarchy are the Seraphim, the Cherubim and the Thrones. These more than celestial spirits are called gods or the sons of gods because they continually behold the order of divine providence. Being foremost in the presence of God, they praise Him continually and pray for us.

In the middle hierarchy are the Dominationis, Potestates and Virtues, spirits of high intelligence, who rule the world. The first Order commands what the others perform. The second steer that which interferes with God's laws. The third oversee the heavens and occasionally perform great wonders. These six orders of spirits are never sent to earth.

In the lower hierarchy are the Principalities, Archangels and angels, who are the ministering spirits who oversee earthly affairs.

The first provide for princes and magistrates, care for kingdoms and countries, each in his own special sphere.

The second are engaged in divine affairs, institute and regulate the worship of God among men, and present the prayers, offerings and pious works of mankind to God.

The third order all things of minor importance, and each one is appointed as a protector to individual human beings.

The fourth hierarchy are the souls of heavenly bodies: Animae Corporum Coelestium, the souls of Hervos vel Heroas, and of the Martyrs. The first control the light and influence the strong, so that their power may proceed from God to the lower regions. The second are the chosen souls of the redeemed. The third are the souls of the innocent martyrs and followers of God, who offered up their lives, amid pain and suffering, out of love to God.

Since God the Father gave to the Son, our Mediator, Savior and Redeemer, all power in heaven and earth, and the angels of the great name of God and Jesus, it flows accordingly into the twelve signs through which it spreads into the seven planets, and as a natural consequence into all other servants and instruments of God, until it penetrates into the lower regions so that even an insignificant herb may develop peculiar powers, and so the angel of man appears before God at all times bearing his prayers into his presence.

Without the name of Jesus, the old Hebrew Kabbalists could accomplish nothing in the present day, with old arts as they were used by the Fathers. Therefore it is that all creatures fear and honor him. All men who believe in him are enlightened through his brightness, our souls are united with him, and the divine power emanating from him is communicated to us.

What Man Receives From the Order of Angels

Man becomes strengthened with wonderful powers through the Order of Angels so that he may declare the Divine Will.

1. From the Seraphim, that we cling to God with fervent love.

2. From the Cherubim, that we receive enlightenment of the mind, power and wisdom over the exalted images through which we can gaze upon divine things.

3. From the Thrones, that we receive a knowledge of how we are made that we may direct our thoughts upon eternal things.

4. From the Dominationis, that we receive assistance to bring into submission our enemies, enabling us to reach salvation.

5. From the Potestates, that we receive protection against human enemies.

6. From the Virtues, that God will infuse strength into us, enabling us to contend with the enemies of truth that we may finish the course of our natural lives.

7. From the Principalities, that all things become subject to us, that me may grasp all power and draw unto ourselves all secret and supernatural knowledge.

8. From the Archangels, that we may rule over all things that God has made subject unto us, over the animals of the fields, over the fish in the sea, and over the birds of the air.

9. From the Angels, that we receive the power to be the messengers of the Divine Will.

4. The Heavenly Powers

The first course in heaven or Mundo Coelesti watches day and night over the world. Primum Mobile Rechet Hagallalim watches from morning until night. Masloth watches from night until morning according to the twelve signs of the Zodiac. From these the heathen nations divided the angels into thirty-three orders. The first great light communicates light, life and station in life out of the first course, and opposes others in the sphere of the Zodiac, causes summer and winter, the spring of all the things which are based on the elements.

Although all things have their source in God, the first Great Cause, we must not despise other causes, such as changes in time, in the year, day and hour. Neither should we regard these causes exclusively and forget God, for in this manner heathen idolatry was instituted. For this reason God does not regard time, because it robs Him of His honor. But on account of the order of things, God has set these causes before us as His instruments, and we must regard them as His noblest creation. We must honor them, next to God, according to their station, not as gods but as creatures which He has appointed as twelve princes over the twelve gates of heaven, that they may admit what they received from the divine name, transposed twelve times.

There are twelve princes of angels, who represent the twelve signs of the zodiac, and thirty-six who represent as many Decuriis. There are also seventy-two angels who represent as many Quinariis of heaven and the seventy-two nations and languages of man. Likewise there are also seven angels of the hosts for the seven planets to rule the world, and four angels who represent the four triplicities of the twelve signs of the Zodiac and the four elements.

Each human being has three angels, for God has ordained that each person shall have a good angel as a protector to strengthen his spirit and to urge and exhort him towards that which is good and flee from that which is evil, fati malignitatem. Every person also has an evil spirit who controls the desires of the flesh and awakens the lusts of the heart. Between these two angels there is a constant struggle for supremacy, and whichever man prefers will emerge victorious. If the evil angel triumphs, man then becomes his servant. Should the good angel prove the stronger, he will then cleanse the soul and save man from destruction. The good angel and his impulses come from the stars.

The Genii or spirits of man who govern birth are joined to each perfection in man. These are recognized from the star which is the Lord of each human birth. The Chaldeans south this Genium in the sun and the moon. Astrologers believe the good Genium comes out of the eleventh Zodiac house, and therefore they call it Bonum Genium. The evil Genium is said to come out of the sixth house. Each individual will learn to recognize him through his own natural inclinations, to which everyone is inclined from early youth. On this account he is called the birth angel who is sent into the world of God.

Moreover God has endowed man with a divine character through the number Phahad, the left-hand sword of God - through which man becomes a curse to all creatures. He has another character in the number of God - Chesed - the right-hand sceptre of God, through which he finds favor in the sight of God and all his creatures. An evil conscience is the judge of men, but a good conscience is his happiness. Therefore through the divine numbers or Shephiroth, and through the angels and stars, a man becomes iimpressed with signs and characters of conscience, which cause him to be happy at one time and unhappy at another.

On this account, if a man has committed a murder, theft, or any other act which his conscience condemns, he can be brought to a confession of his guilt through persistent calling upon the name of God, for his conscience will then give him no rest util he returns what he has stolen or has suffered the punishment deserved by his crime. Therefore, in the name of the Son, Father and the Holy Spirit, take three small pieces of wood from the door sill over which the thief passed in leaving the place where he committed the theft, place them within a wagon wheel, and then through the hub of the wheel and say the following words: "I pray Thee, Thou Holy Trinity, that Thou mayest cause A, who stole from me B, a C, to have no rest or peace until he again restores to me that which he has stolen." Turn the wheel three times and replace it again on the wagon. Nevertheless, all pious Christians, who have any regard for their future happiness, should carefully avoid all superstitious matters and should beware of using the holy name of God unworthily, holding it in the greatest reverence lest they bring upon themselves eternal punishment. If a man knows himself and realizes that he is created in the image and likeness of God, he will acknowledge God the Creator before all things, and afterward the world and all its creatures. From the high spirits, angels and the heavens, man has his portion, and from the elements, animals, vegetables and stones, he has within himself everything that he may desire to obtain.

If a man knows how to discover place, time, order, bulk, proportion, and mental organization of anyone, he can attract and draw that person, just as a magnet attracts iron. But he must first be prepared, just as the magnet must be fashioned by the file and charged with electricity. To this end the soul must first be purified, and dedicated to God through faith. A pure heart and constant joy in the spirit are requisites. He must possess love for God and for his fellow man, and then he may arrive at a perfect state and become like unto the Son of God. It is not given to angels nor to any creatures to unite with God, but only to man, who may, through purification, become God's son. When this takes place, man overcomes himself and can draw to him all other creatures and command their obedience.

But our spirit, words and acts, have no power in magic and knowledge, if they are not everywhere strengthened by the word of God, which we should hear often. We must pray to God without ceasing, live a sober, temperate and unstained life. We must live in a continual state of repentance, give alms and help the poor, for Christ has not said in vain: "Make unto you friends with the unrighteous Mammon, so that he will receive you into eternal habitations." That is, apply your wealth and abundance to the support of the poor, that they may receive their daily bread from you and be satisfied. Christ says: "What ye have done unto the least of mine, that have also done unto me." These are the friends that will lead us to a divine abode in heaven, where we shall receive a thousandfold and life eternal. On the other hand, there are others who will be rejected. For Christ also says: "I was hungry and thirsty and ye gave me no meat and drink, depart from me ye workers of iniquity into outer darkness." Therefore by fasting, praying, giving alms, preparing the souls of the believing for the temple, we may become co-heirs of heavenly gifts, which the Most High will confer upon us in this life if we know how to use them properly.

Since all things have their life and being from God, so the proper name of everything was taken from the being of that thing, and all things derive an influence from the Creator if they have been appropriately named in accordance with some quality of the thing. And thus God led all creatures to Adam in order to have them named, and their names indicated some peculiar quality possessed by each. Therefore each name that has a meaning shows by comparison with the heavenly influence an inherent qualifications of the object, although it is frequently changed. When, however, both meanings of the name harmonize, then the will power and natural power of the thing become indentical. Moreover, kthe celestial office to which man is ordained by God endows him with power to confer life, and tells him what to encourage, what to elevate, what to suppress in his sphere, and to perform wonderful works with full devotion towards God.

5. On the Zodiac and the Planets

As each creature receives its spirit, number and measure from God, so also each creature has its time.

In the Ram (Aries), the vegetables of the earth obtain new vigor, the trees sap, and females become better adapted to propagate the human species. In this sign the fecundity of all creatures is limited and regulated. It has Sunday for its peculiar time and end.

In the Bull (Taurus), all transactions and enterprises prosper so that they may go forward according to the will of God, but to this end constant prayers are necessary, and particularly on Sunday.

In the Twins (Gemini), the angels have power over bodily changes and travel from one place to another through the heavens, have power over the motion of the waters in rivers and the seas, cause love between brethren, friends and neighbors, and gives warning against dangers, persons and objects.

In the Crab (Cancer), the angels rule over legacies and riches, over treasures and treasure-seekers. They are calculated by nature to confer power, the art of speaking, and to enlighten the mind in holy things, as did the apostles in their unceasing prayers to God at Pentecost.

In the Lion (Leo), the angels have power to move every living thing, to multiply their species, to watch, and in certain manners to judge. And through the power of God, they confer upon man the gifts of Physics, Medicine and Alchemy.

In the Virgin (Virgo), the spirits have power to subvert kingdoms, to regulate all conditions, to discriminate between master and servvant, to command evil spirits, to confer perpetual health, and to give to man Music, Logic and Ethics.

In the Balance (Libra), the angels derive from God great power, inasmuch as the sun and moon stand under this sign. Their power controls the friendship and enmity of all creatures. They have power over danger, warfare, quarrels and slander, lead armies in all quarters of the earth, cause rain, and give to man Arithmetics, Astronomy and Geometry.

In the Scorpion (Scorpio), the angels have power over suffering and terror, over which man makes against God, over common privileges. They compel the conscience to obey, and also force devils to keep their agreements with men and **viceversa.** They govern the life and death of all creatures, have power over departed souls, and give to man Theology, Metaphysics and Geomantics.

In the Archer (Saggitarius), they have power over the four elements, lead the people from one far country to another, regulate the changes of the elements and the propagation of animals.

In the Goat (Capricorn), the angels give worldly honors, worthiness and virtue, such as Adam enjoyed in Paradise in his innocence. They also enlighten the understanding and confer human reason.

In the Water Bearer (Aquarius), the angels keep man in good health, and teach him what is injurious to him, make contented, and teach him through the command of God the mysteries of heaven and of nature.

In the Fish (Pisces), the angels compel the evil spirits to become subject to man, protect the pious, so that the great enemy cannot harm him.

6. The Angels of the Zodiac Signs and the Planets

The twelve angels which represent the twelve signs are called in the Apocalypse as follows: Malchidael, Asmodel, Ambriel, Muriel, Verchiel, Hamaliel, Zuriel, Barbiel, Aduachiel, Hanael, Gambiel, Barehiel. The angels also received names from the stars over which they rule as the twelve signs: Teletial, Zariel, Tomimil, Sartimel, Ariel, Bataliel, Masuiel, Aerahiel, Ehesatiel, Gediel, Doliel, Dagymel, which means the same as the Latin versions: Ariel, Tawnel, Geminiel, Cancriel, Leoniel, Virginiel, Libriel, Scorpiel, Sagitariel, Capriel, Aquariel, and Pisciel.

The method of obtaining all kinds of things through the twelve signs is described in many books. The seal of Hermetis teaches how the powers of the heavenly influence may be obtained under each sign in a crystal or a gem. In this way they are constellated. Then, at each period of the twelve signs the appropriate character of each is divided into four parts, each of which is represented by an angel. In this way each of the twelve divisions in the badge of office of Aaron (Solomonis) were constellated. The Amorites possessed a constellated stone for each idol, and to this end they consecrated the book.

Furthermore, King Solomon taught a hidden Almadel or geometrical figure bearing upon the twelve signs, which he called heights. He gave to each height seven or eight names of princes. There are also many other methods of seeking after the powers of heaven in the twelve signs, which for good reasons must not be made known, because they are not mentioned in the Holy Scriptures and were kept secret.

The heights are named as follows:

1. Shamaym   Mathey

2. Raaquin   6. Zebul

3. Saaquin   7. Arabath

4. Machonon

Of the operation of these and their angels, office, order, number and measure, an account may be found in a work by Ratziel, which constitutes the Sixth Book Physicum Solomonis and Elementia Magica Petri de Abano. From this work, the book of the angel Tractatu takes its source. (See Cornelius Agrippa, De Occulta Philosophia.)

There are seven exalted Throne Angels, which executive the commands of Potestates:

1. Ophaniel

2. Tychagara

3. Barael

4. Quelamia

5. Anazimur

6. Paschar

7. Boel

These named with the name of God, through which they were creted, and belong to the First Heaven, Shamaym Gabriel.

The Second Heaven, Raaquin, has twelve lords or twelve heights of angels, who are placed over all. Zachariel, Raphael.

The Third Heaven, Saaquin, has three princes, Jabniel, Rabcyel, Dalquiel. They rule over fire, and each has his subordinate angel. The principal prince of angels in this height is called Anahel, Avahel.

The Fourth Heaven, Machonon, leads the sun by day through some of his angels, and the night, by still others. The Chief Angel is called Michael.

The Fifth Heaven, Mathey, aly Machon, is ruled by the prince Samal, who is served by two million angels. These are divided among the four quarters of the world. In each quarter there are three angels, who control the twelve months. Over these rule twelve chief angels.

The Sixth Heaven, Zebul, is ruled by the prince Zachiel, with two million angels. The angel Zebul is placed over these during the day, and another angel, Sabath, during the night. They rule over kings, create fear, and give protection from enemies.

The Seventh Heaven, Arabath, has for its prince the angel Cassiel.

The angels of the seven planets are as follows:

1. Zaphiel (Saturn)

2. Zadkiel (Jupiter)

3. Camael (Mars)

4. Raphael (Sun)

5. Haniel (Venus)

6. Michael (Mercury)

7. Gabriel (Moon)

There are seven princes who stand continually before God, to whom are given the names of the planets. They are called Sabathiel, Zedekiel, Madimiel, Semeliel or Semishia, Nogahel, Coahabiath or Cochabiel, Jareahel or Jevanael. The planets are called for themselves:

1. Sabachay, through which God sends hunger and tribulation upon the earth.

2. Sadeck, through him come honor and favor, right and the holiness of man.

3. Modym, through him come wrath, hate, lies and war.

4. Hamnia, through him comes light, and the power to distinguish between time and life.

5. Noga, through him comes food and drink, love and consolation.

Cochab, through him comes all trade and commerce.

7. Lavanah, through him all things increase and decrease.

I, Solomon, acknowledge that in the hours Sabachay Modym it is burdensome to labor, but in the hours Sadeck and Noga, labor is light and easy. During the other hours labor is middling, sometimes good and occasionally bad.

Some writers, as for example, Cornelius Agrippa in De Occulta Philosophia, call the seven regents of the world by other names, which are distributed among the powers of other stars, as Orphiel, Zechariel, Samael, Michael, Anael, Raphael, Gabriel. Each of these rules the world 354 years and four months. A few writers believe the angel year to be 365 years, as many years as there are days in our year. Others give the cipher as 145 years. Apac, twenty-one Spiritu Septem in Conspectu Dei Throni sunt quos reperi etima presidere planetis.

The names of the seven angels ruling over the seven heavens must be uttered first, and afterward the names of those ruling over the seven planets, over the seven days of the week, over the seven metals, over the seven colors. These must be uttered in the morning of each day of the week.

7. Invocations of the Angels

"Oh ye aforesaid angels, ye that execute the commands of the Creator, be willing to be present with me in the work which I have undertaken at this time, and help me to finish it, and be ye my attentive hearers and assistants, that the honor of God and my own welfare may be promoted."

Over this there are twenty-eight angels who rule over the twenty-eight houses of the moon. These are: Asariel, Cabiel, Dirachiel, Scheliel, Amnodiel, Amixiel, Ardesiel, Neriel, Abdizriel, Jazeriel, Cogediel, Ataliel, Azerniel, Adriel, Amutiel, Iciriel, Bethuael, Geliel, Requiel, Abrunael, Aziel, Tagriel, Abheiel, Amnixiel. *And each month has her own guardian and ruller, which are described in the Book Of Ratziel.

A person must also know how to divide the months, days and hours into four parts, for God has ordained that all things can best be perfected on suitable days and at proper hours.

The angels placed over the four parts of heaven are: Scamijm, Gabriel, Cabrael, Adrael, Madiel, Boamiel.

Alscius, Loquel, Zaniel, Hubaiel, Baccanael, Janael, Carpatiel

Elael, Unael, Wallum, Vasans, Hiaijel, Usera, Staijel

Ducaniel, Baabiel, Barquiel, Hannu, Anael Nahijmel

In the Second Heaven, Raaquin, the following angels serve:

Nathan, Catroije, Betaabat

Yeseraije, Yuacon

Thiel, Jareael, Yanael, Venetal, Vebol, Abuionij, Vetameil

Milliel, Nelepa, Balie 1, Calliel, Holij, Batij, Jeli

*Note: Only twenty-four names were given in the original work.

There are also four high angels who rule over the four quarters of the globe:

1. Michael rules over the morning winds.

2. Raphael rules over the evening winds.

3. Gabriel rules over the midnight winds.

4. Nariel or Uriel rules over the noonday winds.

The angels of the elements are:

1. Cherub, of the air.

2. Ariel, of the earth.

3. Tharsis, of the water.

4. Seraph or Nathaniel, over the fire.

These are all great princes, and each of them has many legions of angels under him. They have great power in governing their planets, times, signs of the year, month, day and hour, and their part of the world and wind. In the Third Heaven, Saaquin, the angels are:

Sarquiel, Qnadissu, Caraniel, Tariescorat, Amael, Husael

Turiel, Coniel, Babiel, Kadie, Maltiel, Hufaltiel

Faniel, Peneal, Penac, Raphael, Carniel, Deramiel

Porna, Saditel, Kyniel, Samuel, Vascaniel, Famiel

In the Fourth Heaven, Machonon, the Angel of the Division serves:

Carpiel, Beatiel, Baciel, Raguel, Altel, Fabriel, Vionatraba

Anahel, Papliel, Uslael, Burcat, Suceratos, Cababili

In the Fifth Heaven, Mathey, the following angels serve in four divisions:

Friagne, Cnael, Damoel, Calzas, Arragon

Lacana, Astrgna, Lobquin, Sonitas, Jael, Jasiel, Naei

Rahumiel, Jahijniel, Baijel, Sraphiel, Mathiel, Serael

Sacriell, Maianiel, Gadiel, Hosael, Vianiel, Erastiel

In the Sixth Heaven, Zebul; and Seventh, Arabath, over the Fifth Heaven.

Should no Spiritus Aeris or divisions be found, then pronounce in the direction of the four quarters of the world, the following words:

"Oh great exalted and adored God, from all eternity.

Oh wise God, day and night I pray unto Thee, oh most wonderful God, that I may complete my work today, and that I may understand it perfectly, through our Lord Jesus Christ, Thou that livest and reignest, true God from eternity to eternity.

Oh strong God, mighty and without end.

Oh powerful and merciful God."

On Saturdays call upon God in the words which He gave in Paradise in which is the name of God:

"Oh holy and merciful God of Israel, the highest terror and fear of Paradise, the Creator of heaven and earth (as before)."

Quere hoc signum.

PART IV

THE MAGICAL

USES OF

THE PSALMS

The Magical Uses of the Psalms

Or

Sepher Schimmusch Tehillim

A Fragment Out of the Practical Kabbalah, Together with an Extract From A Few Other Kabbalistical Writings

Translated by Godfrey Selig, Publ. Acad. Lips.- 1788

This eminent publisher and translator insists stringently that only persons of a moral character can expect success in the use of the foregoing method.

Extract From the Preface of the Kabbalistic Publisher

It is universally known and acknowledged that we are named after the most holy decalogue or the written law from him. It is further well known that in addition to the laws which He gave to Moses engraven upon stone, He also gave to him certain verbal laws during his protracted stay upon Mount Sinai, where all doctrines, explanations of mysteries, holy names of God and the angels, and particularly how to apply this knowledge to the best interest of man, were entrusted to him. All these doctrines, which God pronounced good, but which were not generally made known, and which in the course of time were called the Kabbalah or Traditions, Moses communicated during his time to Joshua, his successor, Joshua handed them to the elders, who gave them to the judges, from whom they descended to the prophets. These latter entrusted them to the men of the great synagogue, who gave them to the wise men, and so the Kabbalah was handed down from one to the other — from mouth to mouth — to the present day. We know therefore that in the Torah (the Law) are hidden many names of God and His angels, as well as many great mysteries which may be applied to the welfare of man. These, however, on account of the perverseness of humanity and to guard against their abuse, have been hidden from the majority of human beings.

Everything that I have stated here is as clear as the sun, and needs no further proof, and it is equally clear and incontrovertible that the All Merciful God gave the Torah in the beginning to promote the best interests of the soul and the body of man. Therefore God has endowed Torah with exalted talents, powers and virtues so that through a rational use of its powers, man may protect himself from danger when no other help is at hand, and save himself simply by uttering the words of the living God.

That the Psalms and the Torah are equal in holiness and worthiness cannot be questioned. Our wise men declare that "He who will daily live closer to God, who deserves to unite his soul with Him, and who is willing to live in the closest communion with him, should often pray the Psalms with fervor and devotion. Happy the man who does this daily and hourly, for his reward will be great." The Psalms are formed and divided into five books, just like the Torah. **(Editor'S NOTE:** The Torah are the first five Books of the Old Testament, popularly ascribed to Moses and also known as the Pentateuch.) We can, therefore, implicitly trust in the doctrines of the enlightened Kabbalists, when they assert that the Almighty accorded equal talents and powers to the Psalms as He did to the Torah, and that in them many names of the Most High Majesty of God and his angels are hidden, as well as many mysteries.

That this is true, as well as the contents of the prayer with which we end each Psalm, and which we are duty bound to pray, we will amply demonstrate. But its correctness is also established by the teachings of the Talmud and of the wise old men, who assure us that many of our forefathers availed themselves of apparently supernatural means from time to me, to protect their best interests. The truth of this can be established with the most trustworthy witnesses. Suffice it to say that the Almighty has given His revealed true word and unexampled talents and powers for our benefit, and that in cases of extreme necessity, we are permitted to make use of this gift of God for our own and our neighbors' welfare.

Read the treatise on the subject by Rabbi Schimschon bar Abraham in his book entitled, "Responsiones Raschaba." Examine also the comments of Rabbi Jochanan ben Sackas in his Treatise of the Talmud and Sanhedrin, where he treats of magical conjurations, and where he asserts and proves that it is allowed, in dangerous and incurable diseases, to make use of words and passages in the Holy Scriptures, for their cure. You will find similar references in the Treatise of Sabbath in the Talmud, as well as in the Responsonibus by Zemach, son of Simonis, in which the 92nd Psalm, with certain prescriptions added, is highly recommended as a certain means to avoid suffering and danger, even in cases of war, fire, and similar instances, enabling us to escape unharmed from danger.

I feel myself constrained, in order to prevent the unworthy use of this work, to extend this preface by laying down a few rules and limits. Do not, however, feel discouraged at this action, for I am really endeavoring to promote your best interests and shield you from harm.

1. If you are interested in availing yourself of the use of the Psalms, I warn you not to attempt it except in cases of extreme necessity, and when there is no other help at hand.

2. Once you make the decision to use the Psalms, place your trust in the goodness and power of the Most High and Ever Blessed God, upon whom you may perhaps have hitherto called under an unknown holy name.

3. The ordained Psalm and the appropriate prayer with a broken and contrite heart to God, while keeping in mind the added holy name with its special letters, as given by the wise Kabbalists. You must at the same time keep thinking of your undertaking with great concentration.

4. I must admonish you, if you wish to make use of the Psalms, that you live a blameless life without any crime or sin troubling your conscience. For it is well known that the prayer of the ungodly is not acceptable to God. And herewith I commit you to the protection

Further Remarks by the Translator

"Each Human Being," said the celebrated Kabbalist, Rabbi Issac Luria, "Except only the ignorant idolater, can by a pious and virtuous life, enter into the consecrated temple of the true Kabbalah, and can avail himself of its benefits without being able to speak or understand the Hebrew language. He can pray, read and write everything in his mother tongue. Only the names of God and the angels that may occur in the experiment, must, under all circumstances, be written and retained in the mind in the Hebrew Language (for they must in no case be uttered) because, on the contrary, a wrong direction might be given to the experiment, and consequently, it would lose all its holiness, worth and efficiency."

We must all be satisfied with this pronouncement. Therefore I must write all words and names, from the letters of which the holy names are taken, in Hebrew. In order, however, that the reader will understand all names and words and retain them in his mind, I have written all the Hebrew words with English letters, together with their meaning.

I must be permitted in this place to insert another caution. When the text reads "N., son or daughter of N.," it is understood that we must substitute the name of the person by whom we wish to be served, followed by the name of his or her mother. As for example, Isaac, Son of Sarah, or Dinah, daughter of Leah.

THE PSALMS

And

The Many Purposes to Which They May be Applied

PSALM 1

When a woman is pregnant and fears a premature delivery or a dangerous confinement, she should write or cause to be written on a piece of parchment prepared from the skin of a deer, the first three verses of the first Psalm, together with the hidden holy name and prayer contained therein, and place it in a small bag made expressly for that purpose, and suspend it by a string about the neck, so that the bag will rest against her naked body.

The Holy Name is Eel Chad, which signifies great, strong, only God, and is taken from the four following words: Aschre, verse 1; Lo, verse 4; Jatzliach, verse 3; Vederech, verse 6.

The prayer is as follows:

May it please Thee, Oh Eel Chad, to grant upon this woman, N., daughter of N., that she may not die at this time, or at any other time, nor have a premature confinement. Much more, grant unto her a truly fortunate delivery, and keep her and the fruit of her body in good health. Amen! Selah!

PSALM 2

Should you be exposed to danger in a storm at sea, and your life threatened, recite this Psalm without delay and with reverence, thinking respectfully of the holiest name contained therein, namely, Schaddei (which means Mighty God). Then immediately utter the prayer belonging thereto, after which you must write everything together on the fragment of a pot, and with full confidence in the

Omnipotent, who fixes the boundary of the sea and restrains its power, throw it into the foaming waves, and you will see marvelous wonders, for the waves will instantly cease their roaring and the storm will be lulled.

The words, the letters of which constitute this Holy name, are taken from Rageschu, verse 1; Nossedu, verse 2; and Jozes, verse 9.

the prayer is as follows:

Let it be, Oh Schaddei (Almighty God!) Thy Holy Will, that the raging of the storm and the roaring of the waves may cease, and that the proud billows may be stilled. Lead us, Oh All-Merciful Father, to the place of our destination in safety and in good health, for only with Thee is power and might. Thou alone canst help, and Thou wilt surely help to the honor and glory of Thy name. Amen! Selah!

This Psalm is also an effective remedy against strong headaches. The instructions, for that purpose, is as follows: Write the first eight verses of this Psalm, together with the Holy Name and appropriate prayer, upon pure parchment and hang it upon the neck of the sufferer. Then pray over him the Psalm with its prayer. Do all this in humble devotion, and the sufferer will be relieved.

PSALM 3

Whosoever is subject to severe headaches and backaches, let him pray this Psalm, with the leading Holy Names and appropriate prayer contained therein over a small quantity of olive oil. Anoint the head or back while in the act of prayer. This will afford immediate relief. The Holy Name is Adon (Lord), and is found in the words, Weatta, verse 3; Baadi, verse 3; Hekizoti, verse 5; and Hascheini, verse 7. The prayer is as follows:

The prayer is as follows:

Adon (Lord) of the world, may it please Thee to be my physician and helper. Heal me and relieve me from severe headache (or backache) because I can find help only with Thee, and only with Thee is counsel and action to be found. Amen! Selah! Selah!

PSALM 4

If you have been unlucky hitherto, in spite of every effort, then you should pray this Psalm three times before the rising of the sun, with humility and devotion, while at the same time impressing upon your mind its ruling Holy Name. Each time the appropriate prayer must be said, trusting in the help of the Mighty Lord, without whose will not the least creature can perish. Proceed in peace to executive your contemplated undertaking, and all things will take place according to your wishes.

The Holy Name is Jiheje (He is and will be), and is composed of the final four letters of the works: Teppillati, verse 2; Selah, verse 5; Jehovah, verse 6; and Toschiweni, verse 9. The prayer is as follows:

May it please Thee, Oh Jiheje, to prosper my ways, steps and doings. Grant that my desire be amply fulfilled, and let my wishes be satisfied even this day, for the sake of Thy great, mighty and praiseworthy name. Amen! Selah!

If you wish to accomplish an undertaking through another person, proceed in all things as already stated, with this exception: You must change the prayer as follows:

Let me find grace, favor and mercy in the eyes of N., son of N., so that he may grant my petition.

Again, if you have a cause to bring before high magistrates or princes, you must pray this Psalm and the prayer ascribed to it, seven times in succession before the rising of the sun.

PSALM 5

If you have business to transact with magistrates or princes, and desire to obtain their special favor, then pray this Psalm early at the rising of the sun and in the evening at sunset. Do this three times over pure olive oil, while thinking unceasingly of the Holy Name Chananjah (Merciful God). Anoint your face, hands and feet with the oil, and say: Be merciful unto me, for the sake of Thy great, adorable and holy name, Chananjah. Turn the heart of this person to me, and grant that he may regard me with gracious eyes, and let me find favor and courtesy in him. Amen! Selah!

The Holy Name is found in the words: Chapez, verse 5; Nechini, verse 9; Nechona, verse 10; Hadichemo, verse 12; and Kazinna, verse 14.

Still another peculiarity of this Psalm is that should you find, that in spite of all your efforts your business does not prosper, and you have reason to fear that an evil Masal, that is, an evil star, spirit, or destiny, is opposing you, praying this Psalm daily with great devotion will ensure that your business will improve and you will find yourself in more favorable circumstances.

PSALM 6

With this Psalm all diseases of the eye may be healed. Read the Psalm for three days successively, and pray the prescribed prayer seven times slowly, in a low voice, and with devotion, keeping all the while in mind the holy name of Jeschajah (Help is with the Lord). You must believe without a doubt that the Lord can and will help you.

The prayer is as follows:

Jehovah my Father, may it please Thee, for the sake of the great, mighty, holy and adorable name Jeschajah Baal Hatschna, that is, Help is with the Lord (for He is the Lord of help, He can help), whose name is contained in this Psalm. Heal me from my diseases, infirmities, and from the pain in my eyes, for Thine is the power and the help, and Thou alone art mighty enough to help. Of this I am certain, and thereford I trust in Thee. Amen! Selah!

Further it is said: If a traveler encounters danger by land or sea, he shall, when there is no other help at thand, pray this Psalm seven times, each time with full confidence in the mighty and sure help of the Almighty. You must also pray the following: Jeschajah, Lord of Help! May it be Thy holy will and pleasure to assist me in this extreme danger, averting it from me. Hear me for the sake of Thy great and most holy name, for Thine is the power and the help. Amen! Selah!

The five letters of this holy name contain, according to the prayer, the following words: Jehovah al, verse 2; Schuba, verse 6; Oschescha, verse 8; Bewoshn and Vejibbahaln, verse 11.

PSALM 7

When evil persons conspire to make you unfortunate, if your enemies watch for an opportunity to overthrow you, if they pursue you in order to harm you, then take from the spot where you stand a handful of earth or dust, pray this Psalm and keep in mind the HolyName of Eel Elijon, great, strong, highest God! Then throw the dust in the direction of your enemies, uttering a prayer prescribed for this case, and you will find that your enemies cease their persecutions and leave you undistirbed. The letters of the Holy Name are found in the following words: Aisher, verse 1; Ode, verse 18; (according to the order of Al, Bam, and the letters must be transposed), Hoshenei, verse 2; Eli, verse 7; Jadin, verse 9; Jashuf, verse 13; and Elijon, verse 18.

The prayer is as follows:

O Eel Elijon! Great, strong, and highest God! May it please Thee to change the hearts of my enemies and opponents, that they may do me good instead of evil, as Thou didst in the days of Abraham when He called upon Thee by this holy name. (Genesis 14:22) Amen! Selah!

If you have incurred the ill will of an enemy, whose cunning power and vengeance you have reason to fear, you should fill a pot with fresh water from a well, and pronounce over it the last twelve verses of this Psalm, namely, the words: "Arise, Jehovah! in Thy wrath!" Pronounce these four times, at the same time thinking of the Holy Name of Eel Elijon, and of your enemy, N., son of N., that he may not have the power to provoke or to injure me. Amen." After this prayer, pour the water near your enemy's residence, or at a place where he must pass over it, and by doing this you will overcome him.

If you have a case to decide before the court, and you have reason to fear an unfavorable or partial verdict, then pray this Psalm slowly before you appear in the presence of the judge, thinking all the time of Eel Elijon and of the righteousness of your cause. As you approach the judge pray as follows: "Oh Eel Elijon! turn Thou the heart of the judge to favor my best interests, and grant that I may be fully justified when I depart. Give unto my words power and strength, and let me find favor. Amen! Selah!

PSALM 8

If you wish to secure the love and good will of all men in your business transactions, you should pray this Psalm three days in succession after sundown, thinking continually of the Holy Name of Rechmial, which signifies great and strong God of love, grace and mercy. Pronounce each time the appropriate prayer over a small quantity of olive oil, and anoint the face as well as the hands and feet. The letters composing the Holy Name are found in the following words: Addir, verse 2; Jareach, verse 4; Adam, verse 5; Melohim, verse 6; Tanisehilehu, verse 7.

The prayer reads as follows:

May it please Thee, Oh Rechmial Eel to grant that I obtain love, grace and favor in the eyes of men according to Thy holy will. Amen! Selah!

PSALM 9

The principal attribute of this Psalm according to the precept is that it is an unfailing remedy in the restoration of male children who are feeble in health, when no medicines and help are at hand. This Psalm should also be prayed against the power and malignity of enemies.

In the first instance write this Psalm and its Holy Name upon pure parchment with a new pen, and hang it around the child's neck. Repeat the prayer ascribed to the Psalm reverently, thinking at the same time of the Holy name of Eheje Aischer Eheje, that is, I am He that will be.

The prayer is as follows:

All merciful Father! For the sake of Thy mighty, adorable and holy name, Eheje Aischer Eheje, may it please Thee to take away from N., son of N., the illness (here name the disease) from which

176

he suffers, and relieve him from his pains. Make him whole in the soul, the body and the mind, and release him during his life from plagues, injuries and danger, and be Thou his helper. Amen!

In the second case repeat this Psalm and pray devoutly as follows:

May it be agreeable to Thy will for the sake of Thy most holy name Eheje Aischer Eheje, to release me from the power of my enemies and opponents, and to protect me from their persecutions, as Thou once didst protect the Psalmist from the enemies who pursued him. Amen! Selah!

The letters of this holy name are found in the words: Ode, verse 2; Haojeff, verse 7 and verse 16, and in alphabetical order in the At Basch.

PSALM 10

If anyone is plagued by an unclean, restless and evil spirit, he should fill a new earthen pot with fater from a spring and pour into the water olive oil, in his own name. Pronounce this Psalm over the mixture nine times, thinking constantly of the adorable name of Eel Mez, which means Strong God of the Oppressed, saying the ascribed prayer each time you repeat the Psalm.

The prayer is as follows:

May it be Thy most holy will, Oh Eel Mez, to heal the body and soul of N., son of N., and free him from all plagues and oppressions. Wilt Thou strengthen him in soul and body and deliver him from evil. Amen! Selah!

The letters of this Holy Name are in the words: Alah, verse 6; Lamma, Anawin, verse 16; and Haasez, verse 17.

PSALM 11

Whoever prays this Psalm daily, with feelings of devotion, keeping constantly in mind the Holy Name of Pele (Wonderful), and praying the ascribed prayer, will be safe from all persecutions, and will have no great evil to fear.

The Holy Name is in thewords: Ofel, verse 2; Paal, verse 3; and Adam.

The prayer is as follows:

Adorable, mighty and holy God Pele! With Thee is advice, action andpower, and only Thou canst work wonders. Turn away from me all that is evil, and protect me from the persecution of evil men, for the sake of the great name Pele. Amen! Selah!

PSALM 12

This Psalm possesses similar powers to those of the preceding Psalm. The Holy Name is Aineel, which means Strong God! my Father! It is Found in the words of the sixth verse of Ewjonim, Akum lo.

The prayer is as follows:

Almighty Father, my God Aineel! Grant that all conspiracies against me come to naught. Turn away from me all danger and injury, for Thine is the kingdom and the power. Amen! Selah!

PSALM 13

Whoever prays this Psalm daily with devotion, with its prayer, thinking constantly of the powerful name of Essiel (My help is the Mighty God), will be safe from unnatural death and all bodily sufferings and punishments during the next 24 hours.

The prayer is as follows:

Protect me according to Thy will and pleasure from violent, sudden and unnatural death, from evil accidents and severe bodily afflictions, for Thou art my help and my God, and Thine is the power and the glory. Amen! Selah!

According to tradition this Psalm is also a good cure for diseases of the eyes. The patient must procure a plant that is good for the eyes, binding it firmly over his eyes. The Psalm and its prayer must be prayed before the binding, trusting firmly in the assured help of the mighty Essiel. The letters composing this Holy Name are in the words: Ezoth, verse 3; Mismor, verse 1; Jarum, verse 3; Aneni, verse 4; Oweji, verse 5; and Jagel, verse 6.

PSALM 14

Whoever prays this Psalm in childlike faith and trust in the most holy name of Eel enunet, that is, the true God or God of Truth, and prays the prayer belonging to it daily, will find favor with all men, and will be free from slander and mistrust.

The prayer is as follows:

May it please Thee, Oh Eel summet, to grant me grace, love and favor with all men whose help I need. Grant that all may believe my words, and that no slander may be effective against me to take away the confidence of men. Thou canst do this, for Thou turnest the hearts of men according to Thy holy will, and liars and slanderers are an abomination to Thee. Hear me for the sake of Thy name. Amen! Selah!

The letters composing this Holy Name are found in the words: Elohim, verse 1; Maskiel, verse 2; Echad, verse 3; Ammi, verse 4; and Azat, verse 6.

PSALM 15

Against the presence of an evil spirit, insanity or melancholy, pray this Psalm together with its ascribed prayer, and the Holy Name, Iali, which means, My Lord! or, The Lord Too is Mine, over a new pot filled with well water, drawn for this purpose. Bathe the body of the sufferer with this water and repeat the following prayer during the bathing:

May it be Thy will, Oh God, to restore N., son of N., who has been robbed of his senses, and is grievously plagued by the devil, and enlighten his mind for the sake of Thy Holy Name Iali. Amen! Selah!

The three letters of this Holy Name are found in the words: Jagur, verse 1; Ragal, verse 3; and Jimmot, verse 5.

He who otherwise prays this Psalm with reverence will be generally received with great favor.

PSALM 16

This Psalm is important and can be profitably used in different undertakings.

First, if anyone has been robbed and wishes to know the name of the thief, he must proceed as follows. Take mud or slime and sand out of a stream and mix them together. Then write the names of all suspected persons upon small slips of paper and apply the mixture on the reverse side of the slips. Lay them in a large clean basin, filled with fresh water from the same stream. Place them in the water one by one, praying this Psalm over them ten times with its ascribed prayer, thinking constantly of the name of Caar, that is, Living. This name is found in the words of the sixth verse, as follows: Chabalim and Alei. If the name of the thief is written upon one of the slips, it will rise to the surface.

The prayer is as follows:

Let it be Thy will, Eel Caar, the Living God, to make known the name of the thief who stole from me (here name what was stolen). Grant that the name of the thief, if it is among these names, may arise before Thy eyes, and thus be made known to mine and all others who are present, that Thy name be glorified. Grant it for the sake of Thy Holy Name. Amen! Selah!

Second, whoever prays this Psalm daily with reverence and child-like trust upon the eternal love and goodness of God, directed to circumstances, will have all his sorrows changed into joy.

Third, it is said that the daily praying of this Psalm will change enemies into friends, and will disperse all pain and sorrow.

PSALM 17

A traveler who prays this Psalm early in the morning with fervor, together with the proper prayer in the name of Jah, will be safe from all evil during the next 24 hours.

The prayer is as follows:

May it be Thy holy will, Oh Jah, Jenora, to make my journey prosperous to lead me in pleasant paths, to protect me from all evil, and to bring me safely back to my loved ones, for Thy mighty and adorable name's sake. Amen!

Thy two letters of the Holy Name Jah are taken from the words: Shoddini, verse 9; and Mirmah, verse 1.

PSALM 18

If robbers are about to attack you, pray this Psalm quickly and fervently with its ascribed prayer, with confidence in the Holy Name of Eel Jah, that is, Mighty, All Merciful and compassionate

God. The robbers will leave you suddenly, without inflicting the slightest injury upon you. The letters of the Holy Name are in the words: Aisher, verse 1; Shoal, verse 1; Tamin, verse 33; and Haol, verse 47.

The prayer is as follows:

Mighty, All Merciful, and Compassionate God, Eel Jah! May it be pleasing to Thy most holy will, to defend me against all approaching thiefs, and protect me against all enemies, opponents and evil circumstances, for Thine is the power and Thou canst help. Hear me for the sake of Thy most Holy Name, Eel Jah. Amen! Selah!

If there be a sick person with you, with whom the usual bodily remedies have failed, fill a small flask with olive oil and water, pronounce over it, with reverence, the eighteenth Psalm, anoint all the limbs of the patient, and pray a suitable prayer in the name of Eel Jah, and he will soon recover.

PSALM 19

During a protracted and dangerous childbirth, take earth from a crossroads, write upon it the first five verses of this Psalm, and lay them on the woman's abdomen until the child is born, but no longer. In the meantime pray this Psalm seven times in successio, with the appropriate Holy Name of God and the ascribed prayer. The holy name consists of two letter from the most holy name Jehovah He, which, according to Kabbalistical tradition have great power, and which embrace the ten Siphiroth and other mysteries.

The prayer is as follows:

Lord of heaven and earth! May it please Thee graciously to be with this parturient, N., daughter of N., who is fluctuating between life and death. Ameliorate her sufferings and help her and the fruit of her body, that she may soon be delivered. Keep her and her child in perfect health and grant her life, for the sake of the holy name, He. Amen! Selah!

If you desire your son to possess an open heart so that he becomes a good student and learns easily, say this Psalm over a cup filled with wine and honey, while pronouncing the holy name and an appropriate prayer over it. Have the lad drink from it, and your desires will be realized.

Finally, it is said that this Psalm is effective in driving away evil spirits. It is necessary, however, to pray the Psalm with the holy name and an appropriate prayer seven times over the person possessed of the evil spirit. The letters of the name He are contained in the words Hashamaijim, verse 2 and Begoaeli, verse 6.

PSALM 20

In a vessel, mix rose oil, water and salt, pray over it seven times in the most holy name Jeho, this Psalm with its ascribed prayer in a low voice and with reverence. Then anoint your face and hands with this oil and sprinkle it on your clothing, and you will remain free from all danger and suffering that day.

The Psalm is also said to be efficacious in court cases.

The prayer in the last case is as follows:

Lord and Judge of all the World! Thou holdest the hearts of all men in Thy power and movest them according to Thy holy will. Grant that I may find in grace and favor in the sight of my judges and those placed above me in power, and dispose their hearts to my best interests. Grant that I may be favored with a reasonable and favorable verdict, that I may be justified by it, and that I may freely go from hence. Hear me, merciful, beloved Father, and fulfill my desire, for the sake of Thy great and adorable name, Jeho. Amen! Selah!

The letters of the holy name Jeho are contained in the words: Jaanah, verse 2; Sela, verse 4; and Korem, verse 10.

PSALM 21

This Psalm is said to be efficacious to calm a storm at sea. You must then mix rose oil, water, salt and resin, and pronounce slowly over the mixture, this Psalm and the holy name Jehaen. Then pour the consecrated salve into the foaming sea while uttering the following prayer:

Lord of the World! Thou rulest the pride of the foaming and roaring sea, and calmest the terrible noise of the waves. May it please Thee, for the sake of Thy most holy name, Jehach, to calm the storm, and to deliver us mercifully from this danger. Amen! Selah!

The letters of this holy name are contained in the words: Jehovah, verse 2; Duma, verse 14; and Ki, verse 13.

If you have a petition to present to the king, or to some other person in high power, pronounce this Psalm over a mixture of olive oil and resin, and at the same time think of the holy name of Jehach. Then anoint your face with oil, and pray in faith and confidence a suitable prayer to your circumstances. You may be sure your prayers will be answered.

PSALM 22

If a traveler prays this Psalm seven times daily, with the divine name Aha, and an appropriate prayer to your circumstances, in complete faith and trust in God, no misfortune will ever happen to him. Should he travel by water, he will never need fear storms or other dangers. Likewise if he travel by land.

The letters of this holy name are in the words: Eli, verse 2; and Assah, verse 33.

PSALM 23

If you desire to receive illumination about a decision or problem through a dream, then pray this Psalm with the holy name Jah seven times, after fasting and bathing. Also repeat the following prayer seven times.

The prayer ascribed to the Psalm is as follows:

Lord of the World! Notwithstanding Thy unutterable mighty power, exaltation and glory, Thou wilt still lend a listening ear to the prayer of Thy humblest creature, and wilt fulfill my desires. Hear my prayer also, loving Father, and let it be pleasing to Thy most holy will to reveal unto me in a dream whether (here mention your dilemma), as Thou didst often reveal through dreams the fate of our forefathers. Grant me my petition for the sake of Thy adorable name, Jah. Amen! Selah!

The letters of the holy name Jah, contain the words: Jehovah, verse 1; Napschi, verse 3; and according to the alphabetical order Aasch Bechar, according to which the letters He and Nun become transposed.

PSALMS 24 and 25

Although the contents of these two Psalms differ materially, they are equal in respect to their mystical uses. Whoever repeats Psalms daily in the morning with devotion, will escape great dangers and be free from floods. The holy name is Eli, and is found in the words of the 25th Psalm: Elecha, verse 1; Lemaan, verse 11; and Mi, verse 12.

PSALM 26

When imminent danger threatens, or if someone is threatened with imprisonment, he should pray this Psalm, with an appropriate prayer and the holy name Elohe, and he will be free from prison.

The letters of this holy name are to be found in the words: Aischer, verse 10; Lischmoa, verse 7; Lo, verse 4 (after the order of At Basch); and Chattaim, verse 9.

PSALM 27

If you wish to be well and be received kindly in a strange city and hospitably entertained, repeat this Psalm over and over with revrence during your journey, in full confidence that God will dispose the hearts of all people kindly towards you.

Remark by the Translator

Since the author has neither a holy name nor a prayer for the abov Psalm, it may be presumed that its frequent repetition is sufficient for all purposes intended.

PSALM 28

If you wish an enemy to be reconciled with you, pronounce this Psalm and the holy name He, and a suitable prayer, trusting in the power and readiness of the Great Ruler of Hearts, and your wish will be realized.

The two letters of this holy name are contained in the words: Ledavid, verse 1; and Haolam, according to the order of At Basch.

PSALM 29

This Psalm is highly recommended for casting out evil spirits. In such a case, take even splinters from the ossier and seven leaves of a date palm that never bore fruit, place them in a pot filled with water upon which the sun never shone, and repeat over it in the evening this Psalm and the holy name Aha ten times with great reverence. Then with full trust in the power of God, set the pot upon the earth in the open air, and let it remain there until the following evening. Afterward pour the whole of it at the door of the possessed, and the Ruach Roah, that is, the evil spirit, will surely depart.

The two letters of this holy name are contained in the words Jehovah, verse 11, and according to the alphabetical order called Ajack Bechar and Habre, verse 2.

There is no ascribed prayer to this Psalm.

PSALM 30

Whoever prays this Psalm daily, shall be safe from all evil occurrences. The holy name is Eel, and may be found in the words: Aromimdha, verse 2; and Lemaan, verse 12.

PSALM 31

If you wish to escape slander and to be free from evil tongues, repeat this Psalm in a low voice with devotion over a small quantity of pure olive oil, and anoint your face and hands with it in the name of Jah.

The letters of the holy name are found in the words: Palteni, verse 2; and Hammesachlim, verse 22.

Remark by the Translator

Psalms 30-58 do not have any special prayers ascribed to them. The reader is directed to compose a suitable prayer in accordance to his needs.

PSALM 32

Whoever prays this Psalm daily receives grace, love and mercy. With this Psalm will be found neither holy name nor prayer.

PSALM 33

If a man has been experiencing the death of his children at birth, he should pronounce this Psalm and the holiest name Jehovah over oliver oil and anoint his wife with it. The children born to him thereafter will live.

During a great famine, the inhabitants of the afflicted region should unite their faiths in praying this Psalm and they will surely be heard.

The letters of the holy name are found in Lajehovah, verse 2; Hodu, verse 3; Azath, verse 9; and Hejozer, verse 14.

PSALM 34

If you have to visit a high official or a person in authority, pronounce this Psalm and the holy name Pele, that is, Wonderful, and you will be well received and find favor with that person.

The letters of the holy name are found in the words: Paude, verse 23; Lifne, verse 1; and Kara, verse 7.

This Psalm is also recommended to travelers.

PSALM 35

If you have a lawsuit pending involving vengeful and quarrelsome people, pray this Psalm with the holy name Jah early in the morning for three successive days, and you will surely win the case.

The letters composing the name are found in the words: Lochmi, verse 1; and Wezinna, verse 2.

PSALM 36

Pray this Psalm against all evil and libels and they will cause you no evil.

The holy name is found in the words: Arven, verse 6; Mischpatecha, verse 7; and Tehom, verse 7.

PSALM 37

If anyone has drunken so much as to lose his reason and fears are felt for his safety, quickly pour water into a pitcher, pronounce this Psalm over it, and bathe his head and face with the consecrated water, giving him also to drink of it.

PSALMS 38 And 39

If you have been so badly slandered that officers of the law have turned against you and are taking measures to punish you, arise early and to out into the fields. Pray these Psalms and their holy name seven times with great devotion, and fast the entire day.

The holy name of the first Psalm is Aha, and of the second, He, taken from the words Hascha, verse 14; and Amarti, verse 2.

PSALM 40

The principal characteristic of this Psalm is that we can, by its use, free ourselves from evil spirits, if we pray it daily.

The holy name is Jah, and is found in the words: Schauaiti, verse 2; and Chuscha, verse 14.

PSALM 41 to 43

If your enemies have despoiled you of credit and caused you to be mistrusted and thereby reduced your earnings, or perhaps deprived you of your office, you should pray these Psalms three times a day for three successive days, together with a suitable prayer. By doing this you will see incredible things. Your enemies will be put to shame and you will be safe.

The 42nd Psalm is used to discover things through dreams. You should fast one day and just before retiring, pray this Psalm with the holy name Zawa (The Lord of Hosts) seven times with an appropriate prayer. Your wishes should be plainly expressed.

PSALM 44

If you wish to be safe from your enemies, the frequent praying of this Psalm will grant you protection.

PSALMS 45 And 46

These two Psalms are said to possess the virtue of making peace between man and wife, and specially to tame ill-tempered wives. For this purpose, a man should pronounce the 45th Psalm over olive oil, and anoint the body of his wife with it. In the future, she will be more lovable and friendly. If a man has incurred innocently the enmity of his wife, and desires a reconciliation, he should pray the 46th Psalm over olive oil, and anoint his wife with it.

The holy name is Adojah (composed of the first syllables of the two most holy names of God, Adonai and Jehovah). The letters are found in the words: Elohim, verse 2; Meod, verse 2; Jehovah, verse 8; and Sela, verse 12.

PSALM 47

If you wish to be beloved, respected and well received by all your fellow men, pray this Psalm seven times daily.

PSALM 48

If you have many enemies without cause, who hate you out of pure envy, pray this Psalm often, thinking of the holy name Sach, which means Pure, Clear and Transparent. Your enemies will be seized by fear, terror and anxiety, and they will no longer attempt to harm you.

The letters of the holy name are to be found in the words: Achasatam, verse 7; and Ki, verse 14.

PSALMS 49 And 50

If a member of your family is seized by a severe or incurable fever, take a new pen and ink prepared for this purpose, and write Psalm 49 and the first six verses of Psalm 50, together with the holy name Schaddei, upon pure parchment prepared for this purpose also. Hang it around the patient's neck with a silken string.

The letters of the divine name Schaddei can be found in the words of the 49th Psalm: Schimma, verse 1; Adaw, verse 3; and Wikas, verse 8.

Remarks by the Translator

Should someone desire to write and wear a talisman as described in the preceding Psalms, he should procure parchment for that purpose, and a pen and ink used by a writer of the ten commandments. It is said that whoever wears the 50th Psalm as described before, will be safe from all danger and especially from robbers. The holy name is Chai, signifying Living. The letters are found in the words: Sewach, verse 5; and Anochi, verse 7.

PSALM 51

If anyone is troubled by a guilty conscience after committing a grievous sin, he should pronounce this Psalm, with the holy name Dam, three times a day over poppy oil. He should also say a suitable prayer, mentioning the evil deed with a contrite heart. He then should anoint himself with the oil. Within a few days he will find that his heavy burden has been removed.

The letters of the name Dam, through the transposition of the B and M in the words, Parim, verse 20; and Bebo, verse 2, are taken according to the alphabet Al Bam, in which the B is taken for M.

PSALM 52

He who is frequently slandered should pray this Psalm every morning. No special prayer is needed.

PSALMS 53 to 55

These three Psalms should be uttered by someone who is persecuted without cause by open or secret enemies. If he desires only to quiet his enemies or to fill them with fear, he should repeat the 53rd Psalm with the holy name Ai. The letters of this name are the first letters of the two blessed names of God, Adonai and Jehovah, and are found in the words Amra, verse; and Jiszmach, verse 6.

If, however, he wishes not only to be safe from their malice, but also to revenge himself upon them, he must then repeat Psalm 54 and the holy name, Jah. The letters of the name are found in the last words of this Psalm, Eeni, and in the word Immenu, verse 2. This is in accordance with the Kabbalistic rule of Gematria, since the letter He when written out equals six, and can therefore be taken for the letter Vav, which also numbers six.

Should he desire to return his enemies evil for evil, he should repeat Psalm 55 with the name Vah, which contains both of the final letters of the name Jehovah. The letters of this name are found in the words: Weattah, verse 12, and Haasinad, verse 2.

PSALM 56

This Psalm is recommended to him who is desirous of freeing himself from the bonds of passion and sensuality, and who is anxious to be delivered from the so-called Jezer Horra, that is, evil lusts or the desire to commit sin.

PSALM 57

Whoever wishes to be fortunate in all his undertakings should pray this Psalm daily after the morning prayers in the church, with the holy name Chai, signifying Living, which he should keep always in mind.

The two letters of this name are contained in the words: Chonneni, verse 2; and Elohim, verse 6.

PSALM 58

If you should be attacked by a vicious dog, pray this Psalm quickly and the dog will not harm you.

PSALM 59

If you wish to be entirely free from the Jezer Horra, that is, from the inclination which all men possess to do evil, and the sinful appetites and passions which often overcome them, then pray this Psalm from the second verse to the end for three successive days, at early noon and in the evening, with the holy name Paltioel, that is, Strong God, My Rescuer and Savior. Also say the ascribed prayer, and you will soon perceive the most wonderful change in you.

The prayer is as follows:

Lord, my Father and the Father of mine, Mighty God! May it please it Thee for the sake of Thy great, holy and adorable name Paltioel, to release me from the Jezer Horra (from my evil desires and passions and from all evil thoughts and acts), as Thou didst the author of this Psalm when he prayed to Thee. Amen! Selah!

The letters of the holy name of Paltioel may be found in the words: Pischii, verse 3; Elohim, verse 5; Chattati, verse 3; Jehovah, verse 8; Aschir, verse 15; and Maschel, verse 14.

PSALM 60

If you are a soldier and are out in battle, repeat this Psalm, thinking of the holy name of Jah, and say a suitable prayer at the end of each repetition of the Psalm. Rely on God's endless omnipotence and you will be safe from harm.

The two letters of the holy name of Jah are found in the word Zarenu, verse 14, as the last word of this Psalm, and in Lelammed, verse 1.

PSALM 61

When you are about to move to a new house, repeat this Psalm just before moving in, with a suitable prayer, trusting in the name of Schaddei. You will experience blessings and good fortune.

The letters composing this name are found in the words: Schimmu, verse 2; Ken, verse 9; and Jom, the last word of this Psalm. It should, however, be remarked that both the last letters are selected according to the alphabetical order of Ajack Bechar.

PSALM 62

Say this Psalm with reverence immediately after the Sunday evening prayer, and on Mondays after vespers, thinking of the holy name Ittami, that is, the Concealed, Hidden or Invisible (which most probably refers to the invisible God, who covers the transgressions of penitent sinners).

The prayer is as follows:

Great, mighty and merciful God! May it be Thy holy will to pardon me all my sins, transgressions and offenses. Wilt Thou cover them and blot them out as Thou didst the sins and transgressions of him who uttered this Psalm in Thy presence. Wilt Thou do this for the sake of the adorable name of Ittami. Amen! Selah!

The letters of this name may be found in the words: Achi, verse 2; Jeschuate, verse 2; Emot, verse 3; Lelohim, verse 6; and Leisch, verse 13.

PSALM 63

If you have reason to believe that your business partners are about to take unfair advantage of you, and that you will suffer loss through them, and for that reason you desire to leave the firm, repeat this Psalm, thinking of the holy name of Jach. You will then be able to leave the firm without losses and will receive further good fortune and blessings.

The letters of this holy name are contained in the words: Jasjmach, verse 11; and Jechuda, verse 1.

PSALM 64

Seafarers who pray this Psalm daily with devotion, will complete their voyage without mishaps. Neither a prayer nor a name is necessary.

PSALM 65

Whoever utters this Psalm with the name Jah, persistently, will be fortunate in all his undertakings, and everything he attempts will be successful. It is particularly recommended for someone who has a specific petition for it is assured that he will obtain his wishes The two letters of the holy name are found in the words: Joschiru, verse 14; and Dumijah, verse 2.

PSALM 66

If any man is possessed of a Ruach Roah (evil spirit), write this Psalm on parchment and hang it around his neck. Then stretch your hands upon him and say: Save me, Oh God, for the waters are come into my soul. Psalm 69, verse 2.

PSALMS 67 and 68

Both these Psalms contain the divine name of Jah. The letters composing it are found in the words of Psalm 67, and come from the words: Jechonnenu, verse 2; and from the last word of the fifth verse, Sela. In Psalm 68, on the other hand, the words are Jakum, verse 2; and Aora, verse 36.

Psalm 67 should be prayed in a severe case of fever or during imprisonment. Psalm 68, on the other hand, should be prayed over a vessel of water upon which the sun has never shone, in a low voice and in the name of a person possessed by an evil spirit. Bathe his body with the water and the evil spirit will depart from him.

PSALMS 69 and 70

The first of these Psalms should be uttered daily over water by the libertine and the sensualist, who is so confirmed in his evil habits, as to have become a slave of them. After praying the Psalm over the water, he should drink it.

The second Psalm should be prayed by him who desires to conquer his enemies.

Neither of these Psalms have a holy name or prayer.

PSALM 71

This Psalm is said to have the power to free anyone from prison who prays it for some time reverently seven times daily. It has no name or prayer ascribed to it.

PSALM 72

This Psalm will free anyone from prison if prayed by him reverently seven times daily. It has neither prayer nor name ascribed to it.

PSALMS 73 To 83

The 73rd Psalm should be prayed reverently seven times daily by someone who is about to travel in a heathen nation. This way he will not deny his faith.

The frequent prayer of the 74th Psalm defeats bitter enemies and brings them to a terrible end. It will also effect the forgiveness of sins.

Psalm 76 is said to be efficacious against dangers from fire and water.

Psalm 77 will protect against dangers and penury, if prayed often.

Psalm 78, if prayed reverently and often, will confer favors and the love of those in high positions.

Psalm 79, if prayed often, will bring the downfall of enemies.

Psalms 80 and 81, if prayed frequently and reverently, saves man from errors and loss of faith.

Psalm 82, when prayed fervently, will help a business person to be successful in his business affairs and be prosperous in all things.

Psalm 83, written upon parchment and hung around the neck, will keep a man safe from death and dangers during battles. If he is captured by the enemy, he will not be harmed.

PSALM 84

When a person has acquired an offensive body smell, due to illness or prolongued confinement, he should say this Psalm with the holy name Af, that is, Father, over a pot of water upon which the sun never shone, and then pour the water all over himself. The bad smell will leave him.

The letters of the holy name Af are found in the words: Zebath, vwerse 2; and Bach, verse 6.

PSALM 85

If you wish to regain the friendship of a former friend, who is now angry with you, and he is in no way disposed to make friends with you, go out to an open field, turn your face to the south and pronounce this Psalm with its name Vah, seven times. Your former friend will come to you with great warmth.

PSALMS 86 To 88

The constant prayer of these Psalms is said to promote well being and drive away evil. Psalm 85, specially, is said to be very good for the welfare of a community.

PSALM 89

Should one of your own family or a dear friend waste away rapidly due to a severe illness, speak this Psalm over olive oil and pour it over wool that has been shorn from a wether or a ram, and anoint the patient's body, who will speedily recover.

If you have a friend who is under arrest and you wish him to be free, go to an open field, raise your eyes to heaven and say this Psalm with a suitable prayer in full trust in God.

PSALM 90

Should you suddenly confront a wild beast in a forest, or should you be deceived or plagued by an evil spirit or ghost, think of the holy name of God (Schaddei) and repeat this Psalm, and they will depart from you. But you will be even safer if you also pray Psalm 91 with Psalm 90.

PSALM 91

The holy name of this Psalm is El, that is, Strong God. One should say this Psalm and the preceding one over a person tormented by an evil spirit, or one afflicted by an incurable disease, in the name of Eel Schaddei

The prayer is as follows:

Let it be Thy holy pleasure, Oh my God! to take from N., son of N., the evil spirit by which he is tormented, for the sake of Thy great, mighty and holy name Eel Schaddei. Wilt thou presently send him health and let him be perfectly restored. Hear this prayer as Thou once did hear that of Thy servant Moses when he prayed this Psalm. Let his prayer penetrate to Thee as once the holy incense arose to Thee on high. Amen! Selah!

The two letters of the name Eel are contained in the words Jeschuti, verse 16; and Orech, verse 16.

Write this Psalm in connection with the last verse of the previous Psalm 90 upon clean parchment, and conceal it behind the door of your house, and you will be secure from all accidents.

Kabbalists say that this Psalm, when used in connection with the above verse, has the most wonderful virtues, especially if it is combined with other scriptural passages, holy names of angels, characters and prayers.

It is said that through this Psalm all distress, dangers and sufferings may be turned aside. If anyone should be in danger of his life, or be facing any other distressing circumstances, be it what it may, let him confess his sins and then say the Vihi Noam prayer (as Psalm 91 is know), ninety-nine times, according to the two holiest names of God, Jehovah Adonai. Each time he comes to the 14th verse, "Because he has set his love upon me...", he should keep in mind the holy name and then pray devoutly each time the following prayer:

Thou art the most holy, king over all that is revealed and hidden, exalted above all that is high. Sanctify and glorify Thy adorable name in this this Thy world, so that all the nations of the earth may know that Thine is the glory and the power, and that Thou hast secured me from all distress, but specially out of the painful emergency (here mention your problem), which has overtaken me, N., son of N. And I herewith promise and vow that I will not and ever after this, as long as I shall live upon the earth, and until I return to the dust from which I was taken:

(here state your promise to God which may consist of fasting, or giving alms, nursing the sick, burying the dead, or reading from the Scriptures, etc.) Praised be Jehovah, my Rock and my Salvation. Thou wilt be my representation and intercessor, and wilt help me, for Thou helpest Thy poor, feeble and humble creature, and in time of need releasest from fear and danger, and dealest mercifully with Thy people. Merciful and forgiving, Thou hearest the prayer of everyone. Praised art Thou, Jehovah, Thou who hearest prayer. (These last sentences should be repeated seven times at each ending of the prayer.)

Whoever will carefully observe the foregoing instructions three days in succession, in full trust in the mighty help of God, may be assured of the assistance he desires.

Kabbalists, specially the celebrated Rabbi Isaac Luria, have assured us that in time of pestilence or a general emergency, the Vihi Noam prayer should be prayed seven times daily, connecting it in the mind with the figure of a golden candlestick composed of the forty-one holy and important words of this Psalm. (See Fig. 114).

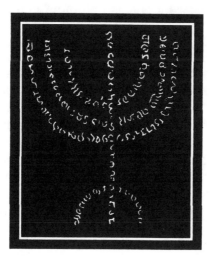

Following are the names appearing in the candlestick in Hebrew characters:

Vean	Alm	Bich	Iba	Wich	Ika	Aan	Beni Ana
Mii	Tmol	Veal	Ktaz	Ilu	Meloh	Imi	Becha
Im	Retak	Betu	Lir	Uma	Ima	Miz	Mehi
Aki	Lakad	Mili	Ibak	Rul	Leta	Afcahm	Pesch
Aab	Schin	Aki	Acchu	Kuck	Vetat	Raasch	Jaub

After this, one should read verses 21-28 of Chapter 12 of Exodus, keeping in mind the names contained in the 23rd and 28th verses, in the following order: Awal, Jahel, Ito, Huj Husch, Aha, Imo, Vil. One should also mention the names Vohu, Uha, Bam, Bili, Zel, Holo, Vesop, and the holy name Nischaszlas.

He who observes all these things to the letter, and who can remember all the letters, points or vowels of the Hebrew characters, shall be safe from all danger, and shall be as strong as steel, so that no firearms can harm him. Kabbalists assure us of this because the letter Seijid or Kie Seijid, which embraces within its meaning all deadly weapons, is not found in the whole Psalm.

Remarks by the Translator

It is regrettable that the reader cannot avail himself of the extraordinary powers of the 91st Psalm as given in this last experiment since it necessitates a thorough knowledge of Hebrew. Since all the recorded holy names consist of the first letter of all the words of the 91st Psalm and of the 23rd and 28th verses of Chapter 12 of Exodus, it is impossible to pronounce the holy name properly. Neither can it be translated into English or into any other language. Anyone desiring to avail himself of the virtues of this Psalm would first have to learn Hebrew. Then he could write the Psalm upon parchment and wear it over his heart as an amulet.

PSALM 92

He who desires to attain high honors, should take a new pot filled with water and place in it myrtle and vine leaves. He should then pronounce over it, with perfect trust, the following Psalms: 92, 94, 23, 20, 24, and 100, three times in succession. Each time he must bathe or wash himself out of the pot, and afterwards anoint his face and whole body with the water. Then he should turn his face to the North and pray to God for the fulfillment of his desires. He will see wonderful things and be astonished with his ever-increasing good fortune. He will also advance from one post of honor to the other.

PSALM 93

This Psalm is said to be effective in cases of lawsuits.

PSALM 94

If you have a hard, inflexible and bitter enemy who causes you grave anxiety, go to an open field on a Monday, place some incense in your mouth, and facing towards the East and then the West, repeat Psalm 94 and Psalm 92 seven times, keeping in mind all the time the holy name Eel Kanno Taf, that is, strong, zealous and good God.

The prayer is as follows:

May it please Thee, Oh great, strong and zealous and good God, to humble my enemy N., son of N., as Thou once did the enemies of our great teacher Moses, who rests in peace, and who completed this Psalm to Thy glorification. Let my prayer arise to Thee as did the sweet smell of incense from the altar and let me behold thy wonderful power. Amen! Selah.

PSALM 95

The holy name ascribed to this Psalm is Eel, that is, great, strong God. The letters are found in the words: Eel, verse 3; and Lezur, verse 1.

The pious believe should pray this Psalm for his erring and unbelieving brethren.

PSALMS 96 And 97

Whoever prays these two Psalms three times daily will cause his family great joy and contentment. The holy name of both Psalms is Jah, and the letters of the first are found in the words: Jeschuato, verse 2; and Hawn, verse 7. The letters of the second Psalm are found in the words: Jismechu, verse 1; and Atta; verse 9.

PSALM 98

This Psalm should be said to establish peace and order between families. Its holy name is also Jah. The letters are taken from the words: Israel, verse 3; and Haschiach, verse 1.

PSALM 99

Praying this Psalm often and devotedly will make a person very pious.

PSALM 100

Whoever prays this Psalm seven times during several days, will overcome all his enemies. Its holy name is Jah. The letters are found in verse 3, and in the word Aetodah, verse 4.

PSALM 101

Whoever wears this Psalm and Psalm 68 on his person, written on parchment, is secure from the persecution of evil spirits and vindictive persons.

PSALMS 102 And 103

Both these Psalms are said to be very good for barren women, who may receive grace and favor from God through their constant praying. The holy name of Psalm 102 is Jah. It is taken from Anneni, verse 3. The name of Psalm 103 is Aha, and is taken from the word Adonai, verse 12; and from Sela, verse 20.

PSALM 104

The frequent and fervent prayer of this Psalm is said to be attended with such great power that through it the Masick may be destroyed.

Remarks by the Translator

The word Masick, according to its root, signifies something harmful. It could mean evil spirits, beings or animals. The Jews understood the term to mean the Devil, and with its connections, the word may be taken to mean sin and the propensity to commit sin.

PSALMS 105 To 107

Psalm 105 is said to cure three-day fever. Psalms 106 will cure four-day fever. Psalm 107 will cure daily fever. The holy name of Jah is ascribed to all three Psalms.

The letters of the holy name are taken from Lejaikof, verse 7; and Hodu, verse 1; and further from Sochreni, verse 4; Tehillato, verse 2 of the 106th Psalm; Jischlach, verse 19; and Verinna, verse 21.

PSALM 108

Write this Psalm on clean parchment with its holy name Vi (two letters) from the most holy name of Jehovah, through which Kabbalists seek many secrets). Hide it in a safe place behind the door of your house, and all your comings and goings will be blessed, and you will be successful in all your business transactions.

The two letters of the holy name Jehovah by a transposition of Vav and Jod, are found in the words: Zarenn, verse 14; and Nachon, verse 2.

PSALM 109

If you have a mighty enemy, who plagues and oppresses you, fill a new jug with new sparkling wine, add some mustard to it, and pray over the jug this Psalm for three consecutive days, keeping in mind all the time the holy name of Eel (great and strong God). Afterwards pour the mixture before the door of your enemy's house. Be careful, however, not to spill a single drop upon yourself in the act of pouring the mixture.

The letters of the name Eel are found in the words Elohim, verse 3; and in Ki Jamood, verse 5.

PSALMS 110 And 111

The first of these Psalms is ascribed to the holy name Jah. By its frequent use a person may compel all his enemies and opponents to bow to him and beg for peace.

Through the praying of Psalm 111 a person can acquire many friends.

PSALMS 112 And 113

By praying Psalm 112, a person will increase in might and power. By praying Psalm 113 devoutly, it is possible to control growing heresy and infidelity.

PSALM 114

If you desire success in your trade and business, write this Psalm with its appropriate holy name on parchment, and carry it on your person constantly in a small bag prepared specially for this purpose.

The holy name consists of two letters, taken tegether from the names Adonai (Lord) and Jehovah. This holy name is Aha, and may be found in the words: Jiszraoel, verse 1; and Jehuda, verse 2.

PSALM 115

If you are determined to dispute with infidels, heretics and scoffers of religion, pray this Psalm devotedly beforehand.

PSALM 116

Whoever prays this Psalm daily with devotion, trusting fully in God, will be safe from violent death. Neither will he be overtaken by sudden death.

PSALM 117

Pray this Psalm with a contrite heart if you failed to keep a vow or perform a good work through forgetfullness or carelessness.

PSALM 118

If you pray this Psalm often and devoutly, you will be able to silence all free-thinkers, scoffers of religion and heretics, who try to lead you astray.

PSALM 119

This is well known as the longest of Psalms. It consists in Hebrew of eight alphabets, but in such a manner, that each letter appears with undisturbed regularity. Through this there arose twenty-two special divisions or Hebrew letters, which are included in each eight verses. A particular power is ascribed to each division, which I cannot present to the reader in a clearer manner than by giving each letter which forms the particular division and its uses. The Translator.

ALEPH

The eight verses of this letter, which all begin with Aleph, should be pronounced over a man whose limbs shake and quiver. If this is done in a low and even tone of voice, he will be relieved. If anyone has made a vow, which has become burdensome to fulfill, it will be easy for him to keep his promise.

BETH

Through the second division, from the ninth to the sixteenth verses, a man may improve his memory, an open heart, a desire to learn and an improved intelligence. Whoever desires to attain this must do as follows: Remove the shell from a hard boiled egg deftly and cleanly, so the inside remains undamaged.' Write upon it the above eight verse, the fourth verse of Deuteronomy, Chapter 33, eight verses of Joshua, Chapter 1, and the holy names of the angels Chosniel, Schrewniel and Mupiel. It is not necessary to know the translation of the angels' names because they must not be pronounced, but they are given here for the reader's information. Chosniel signifies Cover, or Overshadow me Might God (that is, with the spirit of wisdom and knowledge). Schrewniel means Turn me again, Mighty God! (that is, change me, convert me into a better man or woman, as David once said, "Create in me Oh God!") Mupiel means Out of the mouth of the Mighty God (that is, let me attend upon the decrees of the Laws, as if I heard and received them from the mouth of God Himself.) Finally, the following must also be written upon the egg: "Open and enlarge my heart and understanding that I may hear and comprehend everything that I read, and that I may never forget it."

All this must be done on a Thursday evening, after fasting the entire day. The egg must be inserted whole into the mouth, and when it is eaten, the four first verses of this division must be repeated three times in succession.

GIMEL

The division of the third letter, verses 17 to 24, should be prayed seven times in succession in a low, solemn tone and with full confidence in God's omnipotence, over the seriously wounded eye of a friend, so that the pain may cease and the eye be restored.

DALETH

By the earnest praying of this division, verse 25 to 32, a painful injury to the left eye can be cured in the same manner as described in the above verse. Also, if a man is engaged in a lawsuit, or is vexed by a change of occupation or residence, or if he desires to make an important decision or choice, he should repeat this Psalm eight consecutive times. On the other hand, if a man must have the help and advice of many persons to accomplish an undertaking successfully, he should repeat this division ten times.

HE

The division of the letter He, verses 33 to 40, is said to make people refrain from committing sins. Someone who cannot restrain himself from indulging in vices and dissolute habits, should write these eight verses upon parchment, place it inside small bag made for this purpose, and hang it from his neck so that it rests upon his heart.

VAU

Speak these eight verses, 41 to 48, over water and give it to your servant or dependent to drink and your rule over them will become easy and agreeable, and they will serve you willingly.

ZAIN

Two different effects are ascribed to this division, verses 49 to 56. First, if one of your friends is afflicted with melancholy, becomes splenetic or has severe stitchings on the side, write this verses with the holy name of Raphael, that is, Heal, Mighty God, on a piece of parchment, and bind it upon your friend on the site where the spleen is located.

Second, if you are involved in an undertaking that promises bad results through the misrepresentation of ill-minded people, repeat this division eighteen times, and you will find means to withdraw from the undertaking without harm to yourself.

CHETH

Speak the division of this letter, verses 57 to 64, seven times over wine, and give it to drink to someone who has severe pains on the upper part of the body, and he will soon find relief.

TETH

The division of the letter Teth, verses 65 to 72, is an easy, quick, and tried remedy to cure the severest case of kidney or liver complaints, or to take away pain in the hips. Pronounce these eight verses properly, specially and reverently over the sick person and he will be healed.

JOD

If you wish to find grace and favor in the eyes of God and man, pray this division, verses 70 to 80, at the end of your morning prayers, trusting fully in the mercy and grace of God, and your prayer will be heard.

CAPH

If someone you love has a dangerous sore or a swelling on the right side of the nose, pray the eight verses of this division, verses 81 to 88, ten times over the sore, and the incurable sore will be healed.

LAMED

If you are summoned to appear before a judge, pray this division, verses 89 to 96, on the preceding day, and you will obtain a favorable hearing.

MEM

For pain in the limbs, and specially for the paralysis of the right arm or hand, you should pray this division, verses 97 to 104, seven times for three successive days over the affected limb, and the pain will cease and the arm will be healed.

NUN

If you plan to travel, pray this division, verses 105 to 112, which begins with the words: "For Thy word is a lamp unto my feet," a few days before starting your journey, each time after the morning and evening prayer, and you will accomplish your journey safely and will do well in your travels.

SAMECH

If you have a favor to ask of a superior, before you present your request, pray this division, verses 113 to 120, and your desires will be granted.

AIN

In the same way as the letter Mem, which cures pain in the right arm, this division cures pain in the left arm.

PE

The prayer of this division, verses 129 to 136, will cure a boil on the left side of the nose.

TZADDI

This division should be prayed by persons who are called upon to give verdicts of importance, so that their decisions will be just ones. The division, verses 137 to 144, should be prayed three times before rendering a verdict, asking the Judge of All Judges to enlighten one's mind in the decision.

KOPH

This division, verses 145 to 152, is said to cure dangerous or painful injuries to the left leg. These versesshould be said over a quantity of rose oil, which should then be used to anoint the injured limb.

RESH

If you are suffering from a painful boil in the right ears, say the division, verses 152-160 over onion water and let one drop fall inside the ear, and you will experience immediate relief.

SHIN

Say this division, verses 161 to 168, over pure oliver oil and anoint the temples or forehead if you have a severe headache.

TAU

The last division of this Psalm, verses 169 to 176, should be used as the letter Resh, for the healing of boil in the left ear.

Finally, it is stated at the end of this Psalm that whoever is afflicted with a severe pain in both arms, the sides, and in the legs, should repeat this whole Psalm in the following order: 1. The eight verses of letter Aleph, Tau and Beth; 2. The verses of Shin; 3. The letter Gimel; 4. The verses Resh; 5. Letter of Daleth; 6. Letter Kuf; 7. The letter He; 8. The letter Zain; 9. The letter Vau; 10. The letter Pe; 11. The letter Zain; 12. The letter Ain; 13. The letter Cheth; 14. The letter Samech; 15. The letter Teth; 16. The letter Nun; 17. The letter Jod; and 18. The letters Mem, Caph, and Lamed. This method has been tried and proved infallible. Should anyone be afflicted with tearing pains of the limbs, make for him, at the conclusion of the Psalm, knots or combinations of knots in water with the names of Adam, Seth, Enoch, Canaan, Mahalleel, Jared, Methuselah, Lamech, Noah and Shem.

Remarks by the Translator

The translator admits he does not understand this last clause and is therefore unable to guide anyone on the making of magical knots on water. He assumes that no one will be interested in this method due to its complications.

PSALM 120

If you must appear before the judge, repeat this Psalm before-hand and you will receive grace and favor. If a traveler should find himself in a forest where there are snakes and other poisonous animals, he should pray this Psalm seven times as soon as he comes in sight of the forest.

PSALM 121

If you are compelled to travel alone at night, pray this Psalm reverently seven times, and you will be safe from all accidents and evil occurrences.

PSALM 122

If you have to meet a man in a high position, repeat this Psalm thirteen times before the meeting and you will be received with graciousness and will find favor. Also pray this Psalm in Church and you will obtain blessings.

PSALM 123

If your servant has left your house, write this Psalm, together with his name on a leaden or tin plate, and he will return to you.

PSALM 124

If you must cross a swollen streamor undertake a journey by water, pray this Psalm before entering the boat, and you will be safe from danger.

PSALM 125

If you must travel in a country, where you have enemies who have threatened you with bodily harm, fill your hands with salt and, before entering the country, scatter the salt to the four quarters of the earth. You will be free from danger.

PSALM 126

If a man keeps losing his children in infancy, he should wait until his wife becomes pregnant again. Then he should write this Psalm upon four amulets made of parchment, and add to the last line of each amulet the names of the following angels: Sinui, Sinsuni, and Semanglaf. Afterwards, he should hide the amulets in the four walls of his house, and his children will live.

PSALM 127

Write this Psalm upon parchment, place it in a clean bag and hang it about the neck of newborn child immediately after birth, and no evil will ever befall him.

PSALM 128

Write this Psalm upon parchment and hang it around the neck of a pregnant woman, and both she and her child will be safe from harm during her delivery.

PSALM 129

Whoever prays this Psalm devoutly, every day after the morning prayer, will become a pious and virtuous person.

PSALM 130

If you are living in a beseiged city, from which no one can leave without danger and you must leave urgently, pray this Psalm towards the four quarters of the earth before you leave and a heavy sleep will fall upon sentries, who will allow you to leave in peace.

PSALM 131

He who is possessed by the evil spirit of pride but who desires to be healed from this destructive influence, should pray this Psalm reverently three times daily, after the morning and evening prayer.

PSALM 132

If you have sworn to perform a duty and neglect to do so and in so doing placed yourself in danger, pray this Psalm and you will avoid similar occurrences in the future.

PSALM 133

Whoever prays this Psalm daily will retain the love and affection of his friends, and will also make many more friends.

PSALM 134

This very short Psalm, consisting of only three verses, should be repeated by every learned man, and especially by students before entering college.

PSALM 135

Whoever desires sincerely to repent from sin, and to dedicate his life to the service of God, should pray this Psalm daily after morning and evening prayer.

PSALM 136

Every sinner who desires to repent and confess his transgressions to the Almighty, should pray this Psalm beforehand and then make his confession with humility and reverence.

PSALM 137

The praying of this Psalm will vanish from the heart the most deeply rooted feelings of hatred, envy and malice.

PSALM 138

The praying of this Psalm will bring about friendship and love.

PSALM 139

This Psalm should be prayed to increase and preserve love between married people.

PSALM 140

This Psalm is said to remove growing hatred between a man and his wife.

PSALM 141

Whoever is often the prey of unreasonable fears, should pray this Psalm frequently.

PSALMS 42 and 43

The first of this Psalm will cure pain on the thighs. The second will heal strong pain in the arms.

PSALM 144

The praying of this Psalm should be of help in the healing of a broken arm.

PSALM 145

The praying of this Psalm in conjunction with Psalm 144 will drive away all ghosts and apparitions.

PSALM 146

Whoever has been wounded with a knife or any other type of deadly weapon, should pray this Psalm reverently every day, particularly when the wound is being dressed and bandage, to ensure total recovery.

PSALM 147

This Psalm has the same properties as the preceding one, but it also helps in the healing of the bites or stings of poisonous insects or reptiles.

PSALMS 148 And 149

These two Psalms are said to be excellent in protecting against fires, if they are prayed with faith and reverence.

PSALM 150

This happy Psalm of praise to God should be uttered by God fearing individuals after having escaped from a grave danger, or having received a special grace from God in answer to a prayer. The Psalm should be dedicated to the Lord of Hosts with a thankful heart to His praise and glory.

END OF THE PSALMS

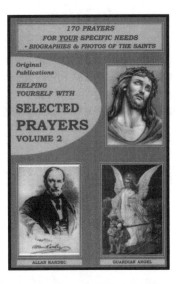

HELPING YOURSELF WITH SELECTED PRAYERS
-VOLUME 2-
OVER 170 PRAYERS!

The prayers from Volume 2 come from diverse sources. Most originated in Roman Catholicism and can still be found in one form or another on the reverse of little pocket pictures of saints, or in collections of popular prayers. Another source for these prayers is the French Spiritist movement begun in the 1800's by Allan Kardec, which has become a force in Latin America under the name Espiritismo. The third source, representing perhaps the most mystical, magical, and practical aspects of these prayers, is found among the indigenous populations where Santería has taken root.

These prayers will provide a foundation upon which you can build your faith and beliefs. It is through this faith that your prayers will be fulfilled. The devotions within these pages will help you pray consciously, vigorously, sincerely and honestly. True prayer can only come from within yourself.

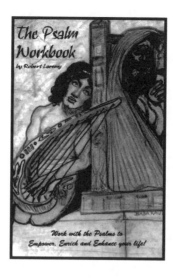

$9.95

THE PSALM WORKBOOK

by Robert Laremy

Work with the Psalms to Empower, Enrich and Enhance Your Life!

This LARGE PRINT King James version of the Book of Psalms contains nearly 400 simple rituals and procedures that can be used to help you accomplish anything you desire. Use the situational index provided to decide which psalm to pray for your specific need.

Peace, Protection, Health,
Success, Money, Love,
Faith, Inspiration, Spiritual Strength
And much more!

Approach your worship with a clean heart and a child-like faith in God's infinite wisdom and you will derive tremendous results from the powers of the psalms.

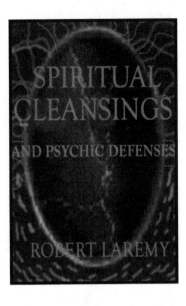

SPIRITUAL CLEANSINGS & PSYCHIC DEFENSES

By Robert Laremy

Psychic attacks are real and their effects can be devastating to the victim. Negative vibrations can be as harmful as bacteria, germs and viruses. There are time-honored methods of fighting these insidious and pernicious agents of distress. These techniques are described in this book and they can be applied by you. No special training or supernatural powers are needed to successfully employ these remedies. All of the procedures described in this book are safe and effective, follow the instructions without the slightest deviation. The cleansings provided are intended as *"over-the-counter"* prescriptions to be used by anyone being victimized by these agents of chaos.

ISBN 0-942272-72-2   5½"x 8½"   112 pages $8.95